Certified Registered Nurse Anesthesia: Critical Care Nursing in the Operating Room

Editors

HOLLY-MAY ROBINS
STANLEY H. ROSENBAUM

CRITICAL CARE NURSING CLINICS OF NORTH AMERICA

www.ccnursing.theclinics.com

Consulting Editor
JAN FOSTER

March 2015 • Volume 27 • Number 1

ELSEVIER

1600 John F. Kennedy Boulevard • Suite 1800 • Philadelphia, Pennsylvania, 19103-2899

http://www.theclinics.com

CRITICAL CARE NURSING CLINICS OF NORTH AMERICA Volume 27, Number 1
March 2015 ISSN 0899-5885, ISBN-13: 978-0-323-35653-4

Editor: Kerry Holland
Developmental Editor: Colleen Viola

Critical Care Nursing Clinics of North America (ISSN 0899-5885) is published quarterly by Elsevier Inc., 360 Park Avenue South, New York, NY 10010-1710. Months of issue are March, June, September, and December. Business and Editorial Offices: 1600 John F. Kennedy Blvd., Suite 1800, Philadelphia, PA 19103-2899. Periodicals postage paid at New York, NY and additional mailing offices. Subscription prices are $150.00 per year for US individuals, $328.00 per year for US institutions, $80.00 per year for US students and residents, $200.00 per year for Canadian individuals, $412.00 per year for Canadian institutions, $230.00 per year for international individuals, $412.00 per year for international institutions and $115.00 per year for Canadian and international students/residents. To receive student/resident rate, orders must be accompanied by name of affiliated institution, data of term, and the *signature* of program/residency coordinator on institution letterhead. Orders will be billed at individual rate until proof of status is received. Foreign air speed delivery is included in all *Clinics* subscription prices. All prices are subject to change without notice. **POSTMASTER:** Send address changes to *Critical Care Nursing Clinics of North America*, Elsevier Health Sciences Division, Subscription Customer Service, 3251 Riverport Lane, Maryland Heights, MO 63043. **Customer Service: 1-800-654-2452 (US and Canada); 314-447-8871 (outside US and Canada). Fax: 314-447-8029. E-mail:** JournalsCustomerService-usa@elsevier.com **(for print support) and** JournalsOnlineSupport-usa@elsevier.com **(for online support).**

Reprints. For copies of 100 or more of articles in this publication, please contact the Commercial Reprints Department, Elsevier Inc., 360 Park Avenue South, New York, New York, 10010-1710; Tel.: 212-633-3874, Fax: 212-633-3820, and E-mail: reprints@elsevier.com.

Critical Care Nursing Clinics of North America is covered in *MEDLINE/PubMed (Index Medicus), International Nursing Index, Nursing Citation Index, Cumulative Index to Nursing and Allied Health Literature*, and *RNdex Top 100*.

Contributors

CONSULTING EDITOR

JAN FOSTER, PhD, APRN, CNS
Formerly, Associate Professor, College of Nursing, Texas Woman's University, Houston; Currently, President, Nursing Inquiry and Intervention Inc., The Woodlands, Texas

EDITORS

HOLLY-MAY ROBINS, CRNA, DNAP, MBA
CRNA Manager, Yale-New Haven Hospital, New Haven, Connecticut

STANLEY H. ROSENBAUM, MA, MD
Professor of Anesthesiology, Internal Medicine and Surgery, Department of Anesthesiology, Yale University School of Medicine, New Haven, Connecticut

AUTHORS

RENEE N. BENFARI, BA, MSN, CRNA
Certified Registered Nurse Anesthetist, Department of Anesthesiology, Yale-New Haven Hospital, New Haven, Connecticut

CHRISTIN BROOKS, CRNA, MSNA, APRN
Certified Registered Nurse Anesthetist, Department of Anesthesiology, Yale-New Haven Hospital, New Haven, Connecticut

MARIANNE S. COSGROVE, CRNA, DNAP, APRN
Program Director, Yale-New Haven Hospital School of Nurse Anesthesia; Instructor, Yale University; Staff Certified Registered Nurse Anesthetist, Department of Anesthesiology, Yale Medical Group/Yale-New Haven Hospital – SRC, New Haven, Connecticut

NICOLE K. DAMICO, CRNA, PhD
Department of Nurse Anesthesia, School of Allied Health Professions, Virginia Commonwealth University, Richmond, Virginia

LARISSA GALANTE, CRNA, MSN
Certified Registered Nurse Anesthetist, Department of Anesthesiology, Yale-New Haven Hospital, New Haven, Connecticut

JENNIFER LACOSKE, CRNA, APRN, MS
Department of Anesthesiology, Yale-New Haven Hospital, New Haven, Connecticut

ERIN RYAN, CRNA, MS, APRN
Certified Registered Nurse Anesthetist, Department of Anesthesiology, Yale-New Haven Hospital, New Haven, Connecticut

SUSAN THIBEAULT, MS, MBA, BSN, CRNA, EMT-P
Department of Anesthesiology, Yale-New Haven Hospital, New Haven, Connecticut

JUDY THOMPSON, CRNA, DNAP, APRN
Director, Nurse Anesthesia Program; Clinical Assistant Professor, School of Nursing, Quinnipiac University, Hamden, Connecticut

CHRYSTAL L. TYLER, DNP, APRN, CRNA
Department of Perioperative Services, Yale-New Haven Hospital, New Haven, Connecticut

SUZANNE M. WRIGHT, PhD, CRNA
Associate Professor, Department of Nurse Anesthesia, School of Allied Health Professions, Virginia Commonwealth University, Richmond, Virginia

Contents

There has been an increased awareness of and interest in patient safety and improved outcomes, as well as a growing body of evidence substantiating medical error as a leading cause of death and injury in the United States. According to The Joint Commission, US hospitals demonstrate improvements in health care quality and patient safety. Although this progress is encouraging, much room for improvement remains. High-reliability organizations, industries that deliver reliable performances in the face of complex working environments, can serve as models of safety for our health care system until plausible explanations for patient harm are better understood.

Intraoperative cardiac emergencies require prompt recognition and management in order to optimize patient safety and recovery. This article addresses the perioperative management of hypertension, myocardial infarction, arrhythmias, autonomic dysreflexia, tamponade, and tension pneumothorax. These complications can occur in patients with underlying coexisting disease, but can also occur in surgical patients regardless of the underlying disorder.

The nursing discipline is vital throughout patients' hospital progression. One of the most critical moments in the hospital stay is the postoperative period. Neurosurgical patients require a high level of nursing care and vigilance and additional postoperative monitoring in intensive care units designed specifically for this demographic. In the postoperative setting, patient care must be transferred from anesthesia to nursing in a manner that is continuous and safe. This article focuses on neurosurgical patients in the postoperative period, the assessment of these patients, and critical care nursing, with emphasis on common issues and interventions for this dynamic patient population.

Massive transfusion is defined as complete replacement of a patient's blood volume or approximately 10 units of packed red blood cells within a 24-hour period or one red blood cells volume in 24 hours for a pediatric patient. This article reviews the most recent understanding and recommendations in massive transfusion along with the unintended consequences in the management of patients with profound hemorrhage.

cooperation with the obstetrician and the surgical team are of major importance in ensuring the safe and effective anesthetic care of this special patient population.

It is important that pediatric critical care nurses possess a thorough understanding of their patient and be able to provide exceptional care, especially during emergent situations in the operating room. This care is accomplished by assessing the pediatric patient, dosing medications accurately and effectively, and performing effective Pediatric Advanced Life Support. Pediatric patients present with unique anatomy, physiology, and pathophysiology. Emergencies are reviewed according to organ system, with a focus on definition, presentation, pathophysiology, management, and special considerations.

Chronic pain is a significant complex problem in the perioperative environment. The management of patients with chronic pain has presented new challenges to anesthesia providers in the perioperative setting. The treatment of pain is often inadequate, and patients with preexisting chronic pain are not being managed properly. Although numerous techniques for intraoperative analgesia have been established, no official guidelines have been published for the growing population of patients with chronic pain. This article provides insight into and awareness of the various elements that should be addressed, along with interventions for the patient with chronic pain in the perioperative setting.

A common requirement for intubated patients in the intensive care unit (ICU) is sedation and pain management to facilitate patient safety and timely, atraumatic healing. The Society of Critical Care Medicine guidelines for management of pain, sedation, and delirium in adult ICU patients provide assessment scales for pain, sedation, and delirium; medications for sedation and pain management, and protocols for weaning sedation, are discussed. Proficient assessment skills, pharmacologic knowledge of medications administered to provide sedation, and an understanding of the importance of nonpharmacologic interventions can help the registered nurse provide patient advocacy, safety, and improved outcomes.

Patients who require general anesthesia to undergo a surgical procedure often require mechanical ventilation during the perioperative period. Ventilators incorporated into modern anesthesia machines offer various options for patient management. The unique effects of general anesthesia and surgery on pulmonary physiology must be considered when selecting an individualized plan for mechanical ventilation during the perioperative period. In this article, the pulmonary effects of general anesthesia are reviewed and available options for mechanical ventilation of the anesthetized patient during the perioperative period are presented.

CRITICAL CARE NURSING CLINICS OF NORTH AMERICA

Preface

Certified Registered Nurse Anesthesia: Critical Care Nursing in the Operating Room

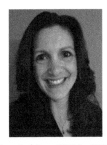 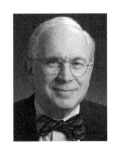

Holly-May Robins, CRNA, DNAP, MBA   Stanley H. Rosenbaum, MA, MD
Editors

This issue of *Critical Care Nursing Clinics of North America* focuses on the relationship between critical care nursing and anesthesia care. Certified Registered Nurse Anesthetists (CRNAs) apply nursing skills that were developed during their careers as registered nurses in the intensive care unit (ICU). In this issue, the authors have brought together topics that demonstrate the application of critical nursing skills in the complex, multispecialty operating room environment. Several articles are devoted to describing the physiologic changes during the intraoperative period. Catastrophic events such as massive hemorrhage and the management of a difficult airway are included to emphasize the skills required to manage a critical event. Specialty areas, including the management of the obstetric patient and the pediatric patient, are included. Critical nursing skills are essential for the CRNA to provide care for these unique patient populations. The need for multitasking in the operating room environment presents a unique challenge for the nursing team. Preventing infection is an important component of the surgical environment, and the role of the anesthetist in helping to prevent intraoperative infection is discussed.

The topics for discussion are not limited to the operating room setting. Articles on sedation options for the intensive care unit patient as well as an article on the effects of mechanical ventilation are provided. An article dedicated to patient safety discusses the contribution of the health care team in providing a safe environment for patients. The critical care period is less clearly defined as technology and pharmacologic advancements allow the patient to move between the operating room, ICU, and interventional radiology areas for care. It is the authors' intention to highlight some of the critical care nursing skills that are utilized in the care of the anesthetized patient throughout the care continuum.

Crit Care Nurs Clin N Am 27 (2015) xi–xii
http://dx.doi.org/10.1016/j.cnc.2014.11.001   ccnursing.theclinics.com

The editors work together as part of the anesthesia care team in a large academic Department of Anesthesiology. We wish to thank our chair, Dr Roberta L. Hines, for her continuing support of the outstanding collaboration in our team and excellent clinical care of our patients.

Holly-May Robins, CRNA, DNAP, MBA
Yale-New Haven Hospital
20 York Street
New Haven, CT 06510, USA

Stanley H. Rosenbaum, MA, MD
Department of Anesthesiology
Yale University School of Medicine
New Haven, CT, USA

E-mail addresses:
Holly.robins@ynhh.org (H.-M. Robins)
stanley.rosenbaum@yale.edu (S.H. Rosenbaum)

Patient Safety in Anesthesia
Learning from the Culture of High-Reliability Organizations

Suzanne M. Wright, PhD, CRNA

KEYWORDS

- Patient safety • Human error • Human factors • Education and training
- Complex systems • High-reliability organizations

KEY POINTS

- Reason's Swiss cheese theory of human error describes errors as results of active failures coming into contact with latent factors.
- It is conceivable that human factors, such as fatigue, stress, production pressure, and situation awareness, are latent factors in clinical practice.
- As a health care specialty, anesthesiology is recognized as a leader in patient safety.
- It is important to maintain awareness of the vulnerabilities associated with clinical practice and evidence-based strategies and thought processes that have the potential to promote optimal and reliable performance.

Over the past 2 decades, there has been an increased awareness of and interest in patient safety and improved patient outcomes. In 1999, the National Academy of Sciences' Institute of Medicine report "To Err is Human: Building a Safer Health System" revealed a growing body of evidence substantiating medical error as a leading cause of death and injury in the United States.[1] The report addresses the impact of human factors and organizational issues on errors and safety and estimates that up to 770,000 patients are injured and between 44,000 and 98,000 patients die each year from preventable medical errors. Medical errors cost our nation close to $38 billion each year; about $17 billion of those costs are associated with preventable human errors.[1]

According to The Joint Commission,[2] US hospitals continue to demonstrate steady improvements in health care quality and patient safety. These improvements have

The author has no conflicts to disclose.
Department of Nurse Anesthesia, School of Allied Health Professions, Virginia Commonwealth University, 1200 East Broad Street, Richmond, VA 23298, USA
E-mail address: smwright@vcu.edu

resulted in saved lives, better health, enhanced quality of life, and lower health care costs. Although this progress is encouraging, much room for improvement remains.[2] The Joint Commission Sentinel Event database lists perioperative complications among documented adverse events that lead to serious patient injury and death. Perioperative human factors with a disposition to error are showcased in the database and include, for example, inadequate communication, incorrect assessment of a patient's physical condition, and inadequate orientation and training of health care professionals.

Health care in the United States is the output of a large and complex system composed of many interacting, interrelated, and interdependent parts. Just as our health care system is a complex arrangement in which health care is delivered, the practice of anesthesia is a complex arrangement in which anesthesia is delivered.[3] An understanding of complex systems is necessary to realize the potential for human error in such dynamic environments. Comprehension of the mechanisms of human error is important when the consequences of a failed system are potentially devastating.

In this article, the most current understanding of human factors, complex systems, and safety principles borrowed from high-reliability organizations (HRO) is provided as a foundation to examine the dynamic and vulnerable nature of anesthesia practice. HROs—industries that deliver reliable performances in the face of complex working environments—can serve as models of safety for our health care system until plausible explanations for patient harm are better understood.

A HISTORY OF HUMAN ERROR IN MEDICINE

Since the early 1990s, there has been a resolute effort by scientists and health care leaders to study the impact of human error on health care outcomes. For example, Leape and colleagues[4] supported the development of a disciplined approach to safety in medicine by identifying and evaluating failures in the system that predispose humans to make errors leading to adverse events. This initiative contributed to improvements in communication among health care providers, such as computerized physician order entry methods, a model that is ubiquitously employed today.

With the publication of the Institute of Medicine's seminal report "To Err is Human: Building a Safer Health System," the state of patient safety at the end of the 20th century was revealed.[1] The report, highlighting a best evidence review of the literature on the potential for patient harm, explores and summarizes recommended changes necessary to prevent and mitigate the effects of injury and death secondary to errors. This publication in many ways lead to the establishment of patient safety organizations, which create blame-free environments for reporting medical errors that may compromise quality of care and patient outcomes.[5]

In the early 2000s, the Agency for Healthcare Research and Quality commissioned the first evidence-based practice center with the purpose of critically reviewing scientific evidence surrounding practices relevant to improving patient safety and minimizing human error.[6] These critical analyses were monumental in creating a list of evidence-based practices for implementation in hospitals throughout the United States. This program, spearheaded by the Agency for Healthcare Research and Quality, sparked interest in examining human error and safety practices in industries outside of health care.[5]

The patient safety movement has generated many promising efforts in improving quality and reducing error, but many agree there is still work to be done.[7] A culture of safety that includes the prevention of error, early detection of error, and minimizing the negative consequences of error is essential to improving quality and managing costs. Strong safety cultures are essential in HROs, where safety is an overarching goal, where problems can be anticipated, and where training and education of workers is ongoing.[8]

THE NATURE OF ANESTHESIA PRACTICE

The practice of anesthesiology, along with such specialties as emergency medicine and obstetrics, is characterized as among the most complex and dynamic professions in health care. The delivery of anesthesia is filled with uncertainty and contingency and is therefore carried out with a significant degree of inherent and undesirable risk. Factors leading to the disparate risk in anesthesia practice include, but are not limited to, the anatomic and physiologic variation of each individual patient, manipulation of the airway to ensure adequate ventilation and oxygenation, administration of rapidly acting, potent, and potentially life-threatening medications, dependence on highly technical and complex monitoring devices and equipment, cannulation of major blood vessels, and management of the precipitous and adverse effects of surgery.[9]

Historically, the specialty of anesthesia had been beleaguered with malpractice claims related to human error.[10] These claims included inadequate patient ventilation and oxygenation, medication errors, and inattention to the environment, to name a few.[9] The anesthesia community rallied around this information and began to address these issues. The advent of innovative monitoring technologies in the 1980s, to include pulse oximetry and capnography, immensely decreased the occurrence of airway mismanagement by providing a sound mechanism for continuous assessment of ventilation and oxygenation. A call by the American Association of Nurse Anesthetists and the American Society of Anesthesiologists (ASA) to remove offending, potentially lethal drugs, such as potassium chloride and insulin, from anesthesia carts in the operating room, greatly reduced the devastating consequences of their erroneous administration.[11] Another example of the responsiveness of the anesthesia community within the last 2 decades is demonstrated in standards of practice drafted and adopted by the ASA and the American Association of Nurse Anesthetists requiring, for example, that anesthesia providers remain physically present in the operating room to continuously monitor anesthetized patients at all times.

Anesthesia providers carry out a vast proportion of their work in the complex environment of the operating room, where a keen awareness of each situation and a high level of vigilance throughout the perioperative period are essential to ensuring positive patient outcomes. Operating rooms are error prone environments where opportunities for egregious mistakes are inherent owing to high cognitive burdens and stress loads, high noise levels, demands on attention, and time pressures. Each day, anesthetists must ensure the proper functioning of highly technical equipment, perform a detailed preoperative assessment on each patient, calculate and administer proper doses of potent medications, monitor the actions of other health care providers as they care for the same patient, perceive and understand individualized patient responses to medications and operative interventions, troubleshoot often ambiguous patient conditions, make complex decisions under times of distress, and respond appropriately and accurately under production pressure.

HUMAN FACTORS

Human factors is a broad term used to describe human performance and behavior and human–environment interactions. The study of human factors deals with a myriad of human characteristics to include the psychological, social, and physical nature of human beings and the system(s) in which they function. Human characteristics leading to error in complex systems include stress and fatigue, production pressure, and lack of situation awareness, to name a few.[12] When human factors are involved in outcomes less desirable than expected, such instances may be attributed to human error. Human error has long been studied in HROs, such as nuclear power, aviation, and the military.[13–15]

Stress and Fatigue

Stress is difficult to define, because it represents a subjective phenomenon. It is generally accepted to refer to an outside influence, such as worry, anxiety, illness, or trauma, causing the human body to respond and adapt in some way. In the early 1900s, the Hungarian endocrinologist Hans Selye developed an ardent interest in stress and the body's response to such, which launched a new area of research inquiry that continues to grow today. Selye described 2 types of stressors: Those with positive effects on the human condition and those with negative effects on the human condition. Under mildly stressful conditions, one can potentially improve performance by sharpening his or her focus and accomplishing simple tasks in a positive and productive way. As one begins to perceive the situation as more difficult, demanding, and threatening, however, performance may suffer as one's cognitive processes are encumbered with attention deficits, memory impairment, ineffective problem solving, and an inability to think outside of the box.[16]

One of the physiologic effects of unmanaged stress is stimulation of the sympathetic nervous system. This "fight or flight" response involves running from perceived stressors more so than analyzing them. When an anesthesia provider is responsible for a patient who is experiencing a precipitous and grave change in condition, this is perceived as demanding and threatening and the sympathetic nervous system responds as it should—by veritably obstructing the provider's ability to think and in fact, encouraging the individual to flee. The trouble is that fleeing is not an option. Anesthesia providers under stress are challenged to defy their own physiology to make timely and accurate decisions to avoid untoward patient outcomes.

In cases of prolonged stress, secretion of the hormone cortisol has been implicated in pathophysiologic conditions such as fatigue. Like stress, fatigue is difficult to operationalize owing to its subjective nature. Fatigue is a complex physical condition characterized by complaints, such as difficulty concentrating, physical weakness, memory problems, mental slowing, decreased reaction time, and drowsiness. Evidence suggests fatigue can have a detrimental effect on performance, especially during situations of high demand.[17]

Production Pressure

Production pressure refers to actual or internalized pressures or incentives that make production a priority over almost everything else. In prioritizing production, the anesthesia provider may increase their risk for mistakes and patient safety is likely to suffer. Production pressure can influence providers to deviate from standard safety precautions and policies, such as conducting a thorough preoperative assessment, checking equipment thoroughly, following other departmental policies and procedures, and checking intended medication dosages and administration routes. Violations of such safety practices pose a serious threat to patient safety. In a hurried environment, anesthetists can commit unintentional errors in judgment as well as performance.[9]

Situation Awareness

Situation awareness is demonstrated as one's ability to know what is going on in the environment at any given moment in time and is ostensibly an essential cognitive skill in the successful management of complex systems where decisions must be made rapidly and under times of distress.[18–21] Situation awareness is a 3-level construct that refers to a requisite quality in operators of complex systems and is defined as their "perception of the elements of the environment, the comprehension of their meaning, and the projection of their status in the near future."[19(p5)]

The theory of situation awareness proposes that anesthesia providers, as operators of and in complex systems, have the ability to (1) perceive what is going on in the environment (1000 mL of blood noted in the suction canister during surgery), (2) understand what this means (the patient has less blood and hemoglobin circulating through his cardiovascular system), and (3) project the implications of such an event (there is a decreased capacity to carry oxygen to vital organs, which could lead to myocardial ischemia and cardiac death). The time it takes for the anesthesia provider to develop situation awareness is crucial because a patient's deteriorating condition, such as profound blood loss, will not pause for the anesthetist's effective resolution of the crisis. The quality of a patient's outcome largely depends on the anesthesia provider's level of situation awareness.

Perception (level 1) is viewed as the most fundamental level of situation awareness. Without perception of key events, the anesthetist is most certain to make inappropriate and inaccurate decisions, causing weaknesses in the system and creating opportunities for patient harm. Comprehension (level 2) involves a higher order of thinking and reasoning to include combining, interpreting, storing, and retaining information.[19] Comprehension describes one's ability to makes sense of the elements perceived in level 1. Projection (level 3) is the highest attainable level of situation awareness and is the ability to forecast, predict, and anticipate future events given the current level of understanding of a situation. In theory, anesthesia providers who achieve level 3 situation awareness are those positioned to make the most accurate decisions and are typically considered skilled experts (**Fig. 1**).[19]

Despite recent quality improvements in the practice of anesthesia, situation awareness remains a key, but not completely understood, component of delivering safe and effective anesthesia care. The concept of situation awareness has been scrupulously studied in HROs. These industries share equally with anesthesiology the characteristics of complexity, dynamism, and risk, yet the study of situation awareness in anesthesiology remains in its infancy. To ensure that anesthetists are best able to perform in complex situations, more research is needed to determine how one acquires situation awareness and its impact on patient outcomes.[22]

COMPLEX SYSTEMS

Complex systems are sometimes referred to as "high-risk" systems. Industries such as aviation, nuclear science, military operations, and even health care have all been identified as high-risk operating systems.[9] Perrow[14] characterizes complex systems as those with multiple levels of dynamic components that are nonlinear, highly interactive, and tightly coupled. Nonlinearity describes the output or outcome of a system as more than the sum of each individual part and refers to the notion that components of a system may serve many purposes. Problems arising in a nonlinear operating environment are difficult to solve and give rise to potential chaos.[23]

High-level interactions inherent in complex systems are described as abstract, unfamiliar, unplanned, unexpected, invisible, and/or incomprehensible.[14] The nature of

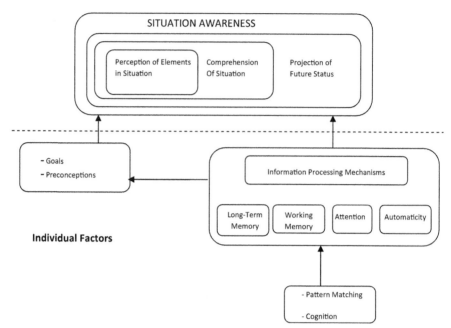

Fig. 1. Adaptation of Endsley's (2001) theory of situation awareness. (*Adapted from* Endsley MR, Garland DJ. Situation awareness analysis and measurement. Mahwah (NJ): Lawrence Erlbaum Associates, Inc; 2000.)

high-level interactions lends itself to the formation of unknown feedback mechanisms and a lack of redundancy, often recognized as requisite characteristics of optimally functioning and safe systems.[14] Orderly functioning of complex systems depends, in part, on the operator's understanding of the dynamics of all components with which he or she interacts and the significance of all types of information produced by and within the system.[17]

Coupling is defined as the association between an action and its consequences. Complex systems are characterized as having tightly coupled parts, units, and subsystems. The term tightly coupled refers to a quality that prevents timely recovery from adverse events and leaves little to no room for error.[14] The degree of coupling in a system dictates complexity. Tightly coupled systems demonstrate strict and invariant sequences, contain very little slack, and demand undivided attention.[14]

ANESTHESIOLOGY AS A COMPLEX SYSTEM

The practice of anesthesia is a complex domain characterized by uncertainty, contingency, dynamism, high information load, risk, and nonlinear sequences of activities at many levels.[3,18,24] Anesthesia providers must effectively, efficiently, and simultaneously control and manage multiple, nonlinear, high-level, and tightly coupled components. These include rapidly acting and potentially lethal medications, indirect measurements of critical vital signs, a chaotic operating room environment, highly technical equipment, and invasive procedures, and the effects of these components on human anatomy and physiology.

In a 2006 study, Kumaraswami and colleagues[25] queried anesthesia providers about the complexity of intraoperative events. The researchers found that patient positioning, endotracheal tube placement and verification, patient acuity, regional anesthesia, and central and peripheral intravenous line placement are among the most common factors contributing to the complexity of anesthesia. Anesthesia is determined to be a high-risk and complex practice in that every intervention is burdened with a risk for patient injury.[3,18,26] In the anesthesia arena, optimal performance requires expert knowledge, appropriate problem-solving skills, adept nontechnical skills such as vigilance and teamwork, and the ability to respond rapidly to deteriorating conditions.[27]

As technology becomes more and more an integral part of a system and the more interdependencies grow between applications, the more complex the system becomes. The advent of state-of-the-art technology such as the bispectral index monitor, computerized charting, and even capnography, for example, adds to the complexity of clinical practice. Barker[28] believes the integration of advanced technology in operating rooms requires essential cognitive skills in the integration of copious amounts of data, in addition to requisite knowledge of pharmacology, physiology, and other operating room processes and policies.

Just as Perrow[14] describes high-risk environments as those that are complex and tightly coupled, Gaba and colleagues[9] describe anesthesia as complex and tightly coupled. At the individual level, patients are very complex with tightly coupled anatomic and physiologic systems. For example, rarely will pathology cripple the respiratory system without a swift and adverse influence on the cardiovascular system. Proper functioning of the cardiovascular system will not sustain itself without quick attention to the respiratory insult. Additionally, many physiologic functions of the human body are nonlinear: Independently, the lungs and the heart are incapable of sustaining life. On a systems level, operating room teams are similarly complex and tightly coupled. For example, should a surgeon inadvertently rupture a main artery during the course of surgery, major loss of blood will result. A delayed response on the part of the anesthetist in this instance can contribute to adverse consequences in the form of poor patient outcomes.[9] In the operating room environment, actions or inactions of just 1 team member can swiftly and very powerfully influence other parts of the system.

All of these factors associated with anesthesia practice conflate to cause information overload that, in turn, adds to its complex nature. The anesthesia provider is responsible for perceiving and comprehending an inordinate amount of sensory input in a fast-paced environment, rich with distractions. Endsley and Garland[19] proclaim that more data, a byproduct of more technology and monitoring systems, does not necessarily mean more meaningful information. These researchers agree that complex systems produce so much data that it is often difficult to find "what is needed, when it is needed,"[19(p4)] leaving operators inadequately informed and cognitively and physically handicapped as they attempt to manage the complexity of their environment. Anesthesia providers, as operators in this complex domain, are not immune to human error and must have a thorough understanding of the nature of their environment as well as possess the requisite skills to function effectively.

HUMAN ERROR IN COMPLEX SYSTEMS

Any system designed to work together to achieve a common goal harbors some degree of complexity and a proclivity for error in the interaction among people, materials, machines, facilities, and procedures.[14,29] A discussion of human error in complex systems is particularly important when consequences of a failed system can be potentially devastating. The study of human error in complex systems such as aviation, nuclear power, military operations, and health care remains fertile ground for improving quality and enhancing the safety of all stakeholders.

The cognitive study of human error is a vast field borne as a development of human factors engineering, which is concerned with improving performance and enhancing safety in the human–environment relationship.[13] Although numerous theories and frameworks are associated with the study of human error, 1 well-recognized and prominent human error researcher, James Reason,[13] proposes a theory particularly appropriate for the study of human error in the anesthesia environment.

Reason's Swiss Cheese Model

The Swiss cheese model of human error describes the opportunity for error as a product of active failures and latent factors embedded in a system's defense mechanisms.[30] In this model, the slices of Swiss cheese symbolize built-in system defense mechanisms where active failures and latent factors are represented as holes in the slices of cheese. When the holes in each slice of Swiss cheese come into proper alignment, a course for error is created (**Fig. 2**). According to Reason,[30] an active failure is defined as any unsafe act perpetrated by persons in contact with the system. These are more commonly referred to as slips, lapses, and mistakes. Latent factors, on the other hand, are described as dormant mechanisms living within a system that create an accident opportunity only when they come in contact with active failures. Latent factors include those caused by realities, such as production pressure, scheduling difficulties, insufficient equipment, fatigue, and improper training.

Reason's model of human error[30] has become a dominant framework for analyzing errors in complex systems such as HROs.[31] The Swiss cheese model does not incorporate mechanical or technical contributions to error; its primary focus is on the human components of system failures because decades of accident analyses expose human error as the dominant risk in complex environments.[13,14,32] Reason[13] identifies examples such as flawed decision making, deficient training, psychological precursors, unsafe acts, and inappropriate responses to situational demands as contributing factors to the commission of error.

After reviewing data from the Institute of Medicine[1] and the National Safety Council,[33] Dekker[34] revealed that "up to 1 in 7 doctors will kill a patient each year by mistake"[34(p177)] where "up to 1 in 53,000 gun owners will kill somebody by mistake"[34(p177)] determining that doctors are 7500 more times as likely than gun owners to kill a person as a result of human error. His purpose for making such an outlandish comparison was

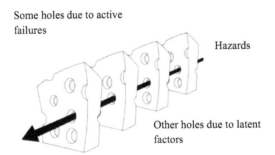

Fig. 2. The Swiss cheese model of human error. (*From* Reason J. Human error: models and management. BMJ 2000;320(7237):770; with permission.)

to showcase that such error counting has long been the mainstream method used for evaluating safety in organizations and professional groups. Dekker[34] explored the Swiss cheese model as an alternative approach to understanding safety in complex systems to support the development of more reasonable error analyzing methods.

HUMAN ERROR IN ANESTHESIA

Human error has been identified as a main cause of accidents in health care and continues to be a topic of considerable importance.[35] Explanations for common errors in health care include, but are not limited to, error in diagnosis, error in the performance of an operation, error in administering a treatment, inadequate monitoring, failure of communication, and errors in drug administration.[1] All of these instances involve some human component. A synthesis of case studies discovered in the scientific literature reveals the impact of human error in anesthesiology. Many studies over the last 2 decades associate human error in anesthesia with lack of attention, inadequate preparation, environmental limitations, clinical misjudgments, insufficient awareness, and flawed decision making, as well as physical and emotional factors.

Caplan and colleagues[36] investigated 14 cases of sudden cardiac arrest in otherwise health patients undergoing a spinal anesthetic. They hypothesized that an in-depth analysis of the anesthetic management of these anesthesia mishaps would reveal common themes in the provision of care that left 1 patient dead and 7 others with debilitating neurologic damage. The investigators found 2 clinical situations to be present during the cardiac arrest incidents. First was the use of sedative medications to the point that the affected patients were not verbal during the placement of the spinal anesthetic. The disproportionate number of cases demonstrating a lack of patient verbalization led the researchers to consider respiratory insufficiency may have gone unrecognized, despite the administration of appropriate doses of sedatives. The second clinical practice pattern identified as common among cardiac arrest incidents in this analysis was inadequate comprehension of the interaction between sympathetic blockade during spinal anesthesia and cardio-pulmonary resuscitation. The researchers hypothesize that a better understanding of this relationship may have lead to more prompt, appropriate, and effective treatment.

Bhananker and colleagues[37] reviewed closed malpractice claims from the ASA Closed Claims database from 1990 to 2006 to compare the incidence of patient injury and liability during monitored anesthesia care versus the incidence of patient injury and liability during general and regional anesthesia. The researchers found the incidence of death or brain damage was similar in monitored anesthesia care and general anesthesia cases, both exceeding the incidence associated with regional anesthesia. The researchers also discovered that an overdose, either relative or absolute, of sedative medications was most often associated with patient death and brain damage in the monitored anesthesia care group; almost one half of these accidents were identified as preventable with better monitoring, audible alarms, and improved vigilance.

Domino and colleagues[38] analyzed data from the ASA Closed Claims project to illuminate the incidence and contributing factors associated with awake paralysis and patient awareness under general anesthesia. Awake paralysis describes a condition where the patient is not yet anesthetized, but pharmacologically paralyzed. Patient awareness is defined as a patient's ability to recall intraoperative events that occurred during general anesthesia. This analysis revealed 18 cases of awake paralysis and 61 cases of awareness under general anesthesia. The investigators used logistic regression to identify patient and anesthetic factors associated with these adverse anesthesia events and found that although patient factors such as gender (female>male) and choice of anesthetic were most associated with awareness under general anesthesia, mislabeled medication syringes and inadequate vigilance were most associated with awake paralysis.

Owing to easy access to highly potent and potentially harmful medications used in anesthesia, drug administration errors continue to be an area of research interest in this discipline. Bowdle[39] examined the ASA Closed Claims database for cases involving drug administration errors. He discovered that during the 1980s and 1990s, 4% of the total database cases involved medication errors, the majority of which involved either substituting a wrong drug for a correct drug, inadvertently administering a drug that was never intended to be given, or administering an overdose of an intended drug. Patient injury caused by medication administration errors ranged from no injury, to minor injury, major injury, and death.

Using a modified critical incident analysis, Cooper and colleagues[40] retrospectively studied 359 preventable anesthesia-related incidents in anesthesia at 1 large metropolitan teaching hospital. They identified a critical incident as an occurrence that had the potential to or did lead to an untoward patient outcome. The researchers found that 82% of the preventable incidents, including breathing circuit disconnections, inadvertent changes in gas flow, and drug syringe errors, involved human error. The researchers also discovered other human factors, including inadequate communication, lack of precaution, and environmental distractions as contributors to critical incidents.

Through a review of the anesthesia literature, Aitkenhead[41] analyzed the epidemiology of injuries and death associated with anesthesia since the 1980s. His meta-analysis revealed factors involved in anesthesia-related deaths to include failure to apply knowledge, lack of care, lack of experience, failure of equipment, and fatigue. Aitkenhead[41] detailed a study by Kawashima and colleagues[42] that investigated cardiac arrest during anesthesia between 1994 and 1998. Kawashima and colleagues[42] described common causes of intraoperative cardiac arrest to include drug overdose and selection error, myocardial infarction, inadequate airway management, high spinal, and inadequate vigilance. Aitkenhead[41] also reviewed the work of Arbous and colleagues,[43] who found that anesthesia mortality in The Netherlands was largely owing to poor preoperative assessment, inappropriate anesthetic technique, poor management of ventilation, and inadequate monitoring. Aitkenhead[41] concluded that, despite advances in technology and standards of practice, patient safety will continue to be highly dependent on human factors, including education, training, attitudes, and persistent audit and vigilance.

The Australian Incident Monitoring Study

One of the largest research endeavors to examine critical incidents in anesthesia is the Australian Incident Monitoring Study (AIMS).[41] The AIMS is an initiative designed to systematically capture information from a wide variety of sources in an attempt to classify anesthesia-related sentinel events. Since 1993, AIMS has recorded such anesthesia mishaps as undetected breathing system disconnections, medication overdose, erroneous drug administration, and problems with intubation, extubation, and controlling the patient's airway. AIMS lists common human factors associated with these critical incidents as inexperience, haste, failure to check equipment, unfamiliarity with equipment, poor communication, restricted visual field, distraction, fatigue, decreased vigilance, and inattention.[41]

The American Society of Anesthesiologists Closed Claims Project

Most anesthesia-related accidents are preventable and involve human error.[27,40,41] Anesthesia-related accidents, although rare, are worthy of continuous analysis and research because of their catastrophic potential. It is important to include the ASA Closed Claims Project in any discussion of human error in anesthesiology because it is a highly regarded, evidence-based, ongoing investigation of thousands of closed anesthesia malpractice claims. Since its inception in the mid 1980s, the project has identified several contributors to loss and injury and has provided the anesthesia profession with effective strategies for quality and safety improvement. Claims reported to the project database have revealed common human errors to include lack of attention, haste, fatigue, stress, information overload, failure to communicate, unrecognized breathing circuit disconnection, mistaken drug administration, airway mismanagement, anesthesia machine misuse, and intravenous line disconnection, to name a few.[10]

The American Association of Nurse Anesthetists Foundation Closed Malpractice Claims Database

The American Association of Nurse Anesthetists Foundation Closed Malpractice Claims Database is as equally important to this discussion as the ASA Closed Claims Project because it contains hundreds of reported cases involving Certified Registered Nurse Anesthetists from throughout the United States. Through a retrospective, triangulated, descriptive research design, Kremer and colleagues[44] examined 84 cases involving cognitive errors that were implicated in adverse anesthesia outcomes. Statistical analysis of the data collected from these 84 cases revealed suboptimal clinical decision making in the areas of preinduction activities, use of technical monitoring, methods of anesthesia care, and preventability of a damaging event.

Holden[45] suggests that a focus on the thought processes and behaviors of individuals and the systems in which they work, rather than on the attribution of error, may be among the most productive methods for reducing the catastrophic potential intrinsic to complex systems. Similarly, the work of Reason[13] proposes that, to understand human error in complex systems, further empirical attention should be directed toward the cognitive aspects of human behavior rather than on errors themselves.

ANESTHESIA CRISIS RESOURCE MANAGEMENT AND SIMULATION TRAINING

Simulation involves the implementation of artificial representations of complex, real-world processes through a sufficient level of fidelity to achieve training and educational goals. Simulation is an innovative instructional approach to enriching the climate for learning and promoting a sense of empowerment on the part of learners by actively engaging them as much as possible. Through simulation, trainees can be challenged in ways previously not possible, taking more responsibility in their learning. A critical feature of simulation as an effective teaching tool is the student's ability to interact with the environment experimentally, as opposed to only observing it.

Simulation training has a rich history in HROs, such as aviation and air traffic control, the military, and nuclear power—industries where the propensity for error is high and such errors can be catastrophic. Only recently has the use of simulation been integrated into the training of health care professionals. Using high-fidelity simulated environments, educators can create clinically relevant crises in an environment of chaos where the risk to a real patient is naught.

Anesthesia Crisis Resource Management (ACRM) training was adapted from the aviation industry's Crew Resource Management training for pilots and crews.[9] Crew Resource Management training programs resulted from the realization that, despite adequate simulation training addressing technical skills, airline pilots were ill-equipped with the essential management skills required to manage the critical and unexpected events implicated in most airline disasters. Likewise, the delivery of safe anesthesia care involves more than subject matter knowledge and technical skills, such as endotracheal intubation, central line placement, and regional anesthesia. Instead, knowledge and technical skills must be assimilated into practice through the employ of proficient nontechnical skills.

ACRM training incorporates human patient simulators in high-fidelity operating room environments to simulate rare but life-threatening anesthesia crises, including malignant hyperthermia, pulmonary embolism, inability to ventilate, anaphylactic shock, and cardiac arrest. Human patient simulators, sometimes referred to as mannequins, are full-body representations of patients that demonstrate physiologic parameters, such as blood pressure, heart rate, airway pressure, oxygen saturation, and central venous and pulmonary pressure. Different models of human patient simulators offer varying degrees of realism, including bleeding, sweating, pupil constriction and dilation, seizures, chest movement, and peripheral pulses. Human patient simulators are supported by software that is operated by a controller behind 1-way glass. The controller can steer the human patient simulator to respond to trainee interventions, such as medication and fluid administration, defibrillation, chest tube insertion, and oxygenation. Human patient simulators are highly effective in contributing to the fidelity necessary to simulate a real operating room environment.

ACRM emphasizes the integration of principles of crisis management, including decision making, task management, leadership, communication, situation awareness, and teamwork, in training anesthesia providers with wide ranges of experience to manage critical events and crisis situations. Identifying and mastering ideal case management thoughts and behaviors, including preparation, anticipation, and vigilance, are also a major goal of ACRM training. Factors such as production pressure, problem solving, decision making, and abstract reasoning and their influence on the provider to act optimally and reliably are considered and explored.

ACRM is an experiential teaching approach that brings the daunting characteristics of an anesthesia crisis to life and ultimately aims to improve efficiency, effectiveness, and safety in the delivery of anesthesia. Most ACRM courses have a similar structure that incorporates assigned readings describing basic safety principles, a course introduction detailing the overall conceptual view of ACRM training, and an orientation to the simulated operating room environment and human patient simulator. During ACRM training, the trainee is an active participant carrying out the duties of the anesthesia provider under the extreme conditions of an anesthetic emergency (**Fig. 3**).

A video playback and directed debriefing session immediately follow the scenario. Debriefing is a discussion among trainees, guided by the course instructor, that encourages reflective thought and self-review. Debriefing is regarded as an integral part of ACRM and occurs in a positive, supportive, nonjudgmental and nonevaluative environment that allows all participants an opportunity to share their experience, offer comments, and discuss concerns.

Alternatively, anesthesia crisis management training depends on the standard teaching model of didactic instruction, assigned readings, and apprenticeship during clinical rotations under the watchful eye of a preceptor with real patients in real

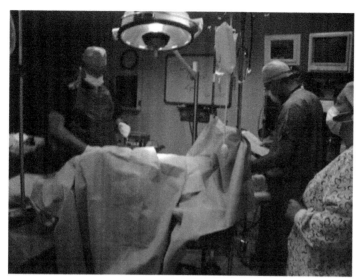

Fig. 3. Graduate nurse anesthesia student participating in anesthesia crisis resource management (ACRM) in a high-fidelity simulated operation room environment. (*Courtesy of* Center for Research in Human Simulation, Department of Nurse Anesthesia, Virginia Commonwealth University, Richmond, Virginia.

operating rooms. One disadvantage to this approach is that it may support the inculcation and regurgitation of information that often results in no clinical application of the same. Furthermore, the likelihood of life-threatening anesthesia crises actually occurring frequently enough to sufficiently train anesthetists adequately is remote and inconsistent at best. If a life-threatening anesthesia crisis does occur under the clinical apprenticeship model, it is likely that learning will take place. It may do so, however, without a solid grounding in theory or the basic principles of ACRM, thereby potentially minimizing the long-lasting impact of the experience. Developing such complex crisis management behaviors such as those required to work effectively in teams or to communicate effectively requires more than a 1- or 2-time simulation training exercise. These behaviors grow over time by continued practice and reinforcement.

SUMMARY

In an effort to improve quality and safety in complex systems, many industries have examined the impact of human factors. Much of the existing literature on human factors and safety comes from HROs, such as aviation, air traffic control, and military operations, with most seminal articles dating back to the 1990s. Given the limited research of human factors in anesthesiology, work was done in this article to share evidence of a significant link between human error and complex systems and complex systems and anesthesiology to communicate a need for further study of these areas in an effort to improve patient safety.

Reason's Swiss Cheese theory of human error[13] describes errors as results of active failures, also named triggers, coming into contact with latent factors; dormant and faulty mechanisms living within a system. Reason[13] provides examples of latent factors as fatigue, improper training, and scheduling problems. It is conceivable that human factors such as fatigue, stress, production pressure, and situation awareness may serve as latent factors in clinical practice.

As a health care specialty, anesthesiology is recognized as a leader in patient safety. It is important, however, to maintain continuous awareness of the vulnerabilities associated with clinical practice as well as evidence-based strategies and thought processes that have the potential to promote optimal and reliable performance. Until error, adverse outcomes, and patient harm are better understood and the incidence of such is greatly and reliably reduced, we owe it to ourselves and to our patients to continue to entertain all possible explanations for these unexpected and undesirable events.

REFERENCES

1. Kohn LT, Corrigan JM, Donaldson M, editors. To err is human: building a safer health system. Washington, DC: Institute of Medicine; 1999.
2. The Joint Commission. Improving America's Hospitals: The Joint Commission's Annual Report on Quality and Safety. The Joint Commission. 2007. Available at: http://www.jointcommissionreport.org/pdf/JC_2007_Annual_Report.pdf. Accessed August 20, 2008.
3. Pott C, Johnson A, Cnossen F. Improving situation awareness in anaesthesiology. Proceedings of the 2005 Annual Conference on European Association of Cognitive Ergonomics. vol. 132. Athens (Greece): University of Athens; 2005. p. 255–63.
4. Leape LL, Bates DW, Cullen DJ, et al. Systems analysis of adverse drug events. ADE Prevention Study Group. JAMA 1995;274:35–43.
5. Ilan RI, Fowler R. Brief history of patient safety culture and science. J Crit Care 2005;20:2–5.
6. Shojania KG, Duncan BW, McDonald KM. Making health care safer: a critical analysis of patient safety practices. Rockville (MD): Agency for Healthcare and Research Quality; 2001.
7. Altman DE, Clancy C, Blendon RJ. Improving patient safety – five years after the IOM report. N Engl J Med 2004;351(20):2041–3.
8. Benhamou D, Auroy Y, Amalberti R. Monitoring quality and safety in anesthesia: are large numbers enough? Anesth Analg 2007;107(5):1458–60.
9. Gaba DM, Fish KJ, Howard SK. Theory of dynamic decision making and crisis management. Crisis management in anesthesiology. New York: Churchill Livingstone, Inc; 1994. p. 5–46.
10. Cheney FW. The American Society of Anesthesiologists Closed Claims Project: what have we learned, how has it affected practice and how will it affect practice in the future? Anesthesiology 1999;91(2):552–6.
11. US Pharmacopeia. USP quality review. 2000. Available at: http://www.usp.org/pdf/EN/patientSafety/pSafetySMUExpCommArticle.pdf. Accessed December 10, 2008.
12. Whittingham RB. The blame machine: why human error causes accidents. Burlington (MA): Elsevier Butterworth-Heinemann; 2004.
13. Reason J. Human error. New York: Cambridge University Press; 1990.
14. Perrow C. Normal accidents: living with high-risk technologies. Princeton (NJ): Princeton University Press; 1999.
15. Sheridan TB. Human error. Qual Saf Health Care 2003;12(5):383–5.
16. Eisner H. Managing complex systems: thinking outside the box. Hoboken (NJ): John Wiley & Sons, Inc; 2005.
17. Cannon-Bowers JA, Salas E. Making decisions under stress: implications for training. Washington, DC: American Psychological Association; 2006.

18. Gaba DM, Howard SK. Situation awareness in anesthesiology. Hum Factors 1995;37(1):20–31.
19. Endsley MR, Garland DJ. Situation awareness analysis and measurement. Mahwah (NJ): Lawrence Erlbaum Associates, Inc; 2000.
20. Wright MC, Taekman JM, Endsley MR. Objective measures of situation awareness in a simulated medical environment. Qual Saf Health Care 2004;13:65–71.
21. McIlvaine WB. Situational awareness in the operating room: a primer for the anesthesiologist. Semin Anesth Perioper Med Pain 2007;26(3):167–72.
22. Kogan MJ. Human factors viewed as key to reducing medical errors. Mon Psychol 2000;31(11). p. 29. Available at: http://www.apa.org/monitor/dec00/human.html. Accessed December 19, 2008.
23. Khalil HK. Nonlinear systems. Upper Saddle River (NJ): Prentice-Hall; 2001.
24. Runciman B, Merry A, Walton R. Safety and ethics in healthcare: a guide to getting it right. Burlington (VT): Ashgate Publishing Limited; 2007.
25. Kumaraswami MB, Holt NF, Senior A, et al. Factors that increase anesthetic complexity: can we address them? Anesthesiology 2006;105:A1306.
26. Wright M. Time of day effects on the incidence of anesthetic adverse events. Qual Saf Health Care 2006;15(4):258–63.
27. Weinger MB, Slagle JS. Human factors research in anesthesia patient safety. J Am Med Inform Assn 2002;9(6 Suppl 1):58–63.
28. Barker T. Too much technology? Anesth Analg 2003;97(4):938–9.
29. Chapanis A. Human factors in system engineering. New York: John Wiley and Sons; 1996.
30. Reason J. Human error: models and management. BMJ 2000;320(7237): 768–70.
31. Perneger TV. The Swiss cheese model of safety incidents: are there holes in the metaphor? BMC Health Serv Res 2005;5:71.
32. Strauch B. Investigating human error: incidents, accidents, and complex systems. Burlington (VT): Ashgate Publishing Limited; 2004.
33. National Safety Council. Injury facts, 2004 edition. Itasca (IL): National Safety Council; 2004.
34. Dekker SW. Doctors are more dangerous than gun owners: a rejoinder to error counting. Hum Factors 2007;49(2):177–84.
35. Nyssen AS, Blavier A. Error detection: a study in anaesthesia. Ergonomics 2006; 49(5):517–25.
36. Caplan RA, Ward RJ, Posner KB, et al. Unexpected cardiac arrest during spinal anesthesia: a closed claims analysis of predisposing factors. Anesthesiology 1988;68(1):5–11.
37. Bhananker SM, Posner KL, Cheney FW, et al. Injury and liability associated with monitored anesthesia care. Anesthesiology 2006;104(2):228–34.
38. Domino KB, Posner KL, Caplan RA, et al. Awareness during anesthesia. Anesthesiology 1999;90(4):1053.
39. Bowdle TA. Drug administration errors from the ASA closed claims project. ASA Newsl 2003;67(6):11–3.
40. Cooper J, Newbower C, McPeek B. Preventable anesthesia mishaps: a study of human factors. Qual Saf Health Care 2002;11(3):277–82.
41. Aitkenhead AR. Injuries associated with anesthesia: a global perspective. Br J Anaesth 2005;95(1):95–109.
42. Kawashima Y, Takahashi S, Suzuki M, et al. Anesthesia-related mortality and morbidity over a 5-year period in 2,363,038 patients in Japan. Acta Anaesthesiol Scand 2003;47(7):809–17.

43. Arbous MS, Meursing AE, van Kleef JW, et al. Impact of anesthesia management characteristics on severe morbidity and mortality. Anesthesiology 2005;102: 257–68.
44. Kremer MJ, Faut-Callahan M, Hicks FD. A study of clinical decision making by certified registered nurse anesthetists. AANA J 2002;70(5):391–7.
45. Holden R. People or systems? To blame is human. The fix is to engineer. Prof Saf 2009;54(12):34–41.

Intraoperative Cardiac Emergencies

Chrystal L. Tyler, DNP, APRN, CRNA

KEYWORDS

- Perioperative hypertension • Myocardial infarction • Arrhythmias
- Autonomic dysreflexia • Tension pneumothorax • Tamponade

KEY POINTS

- Thorough preoperative evaluation and assessment of cardiac risk allows the anticipation of intraoperative cardiac alterations.
- Hypertension is a common coexisting disease of surgical patients and can exacerbate during the intraoperative period. Maintenance of the patient's baseline hemodynamics and pharmacologic treatment can optimize outcomes for these patients.
- There are various cardiac emergencies that can occur perioperatively, all requiring an astute practitioner for rapid assessment and treatment to decrease the associated morbidity and mortality.

INTRODUCTION

Cardiac complications constitute the most common cause of postoperative morbidity and mortality, strongly affecting the length and cost of hospitalization.[1] Cardiac alterations that present perioperatively include hypertension, myocardial infarction (MI) or ischemia, arrhythmias, autonomic dysreflexia, tension pneumothorax, and tamponade. Cardiac complications of death, MI, heart failure, or ventricular tachycardia occur in up to 5% of patients aged 45 years and older undergoing in-hospital noncardiac surgery.[2] Of these, perioperative MI is the most common. Thorough preoperative evaluations are necessary to clarify a patient's cardiac risk associated with the individual surgery presented. Certified Registered Nurse Anesthetists are directly involved in the assessment, management, and recovery of these patients during the perioperative period. Optimal outcomes from cardiac emergencies begin with prompt recognition and keen assessment to identify a change in a patient's status.

The author has nothing to disclose.
Department of Perioperative Services, Yale-New Haven Hospital, 20 York Street, New Haven, CT 06510, USA
E-mail address: ctyler706@gmail.com

Crit Care Nurs Clin N Am 27 (2015) 17–31
http://dx.doi.org/10.1016/j.cnc.2014.10.009   ccnursing.theclinics.com

HYPERTENSION

Hypertension is a commonly encountered coexisting disease in surgical patients. It affects roughly 30% of the United States population more than 18 years old and is one of the most common chronic medical conditions.[3] In individuals older than 65 years, two-thirds of the population have hypertension.[4] Hypertension is a strong risk factor for coronary artery disease (CAD) and also a cause of congestive heart failure and cardiomyopathy caused by the increased afterload from chronic vasoconstriction.[4] Hypertension is a risk factor for complications following anesthesia and surgery. Considering the prevalence of hypertension, the strict and thorough management of these patients undergoing surgery is critical to avoiding the associated morbidity and mortality.

Table 1 describes the different classifications of blood pressure. The Seventh Report of the Joint National Committee defined hypertensive crisis as systolic blood pressure greater than 180 mm Hg or a diastolic blood pressure greater than 110 mm Hg.[5] Hypertensive crisis in the perioperative setting usually presents in patients who are untreated or inadequately treated.[6] This term encompasses both hypertensive emergencies and urgencies, which are differentiated as follows:

- Hypertensive emergency: severe increase in blood pressure complicated by evidence of progressive organ dysfunction. This condition requires immediate blood pressure reduction to limit organ damage.
- Hypertensive urgency: severe increase in blood pressure without organ dysfunction.

Patients who are optimized before surgery have a more stable intraoperative course,[4] therefore it is essential to include certain details in the preoperative assessment:

- Clarify whether the patient has been on an adequate treatment regimen (determine the last dose of medications)
- Determine the level at which the patient's blood pressure is usually maintained
- Because hypertension is a major risk factor for CAD, evaluate the patient for any signs of ischemia

The decision to cancel elective surgery for preoperative hypertension is controversial and varies with practitioner experience and judgment. Wax and colleagues[7] performed a retrospective analysis to investigate the incidence of preoperative hypertension, case cancellations, and association with postoperative outcomes. The severity of preinduction hypertension was an independent risk factor for postoperative myocardial injury/infarction or in-hospital death. However, the small percentage of

Table 1 Classifications of blood pressure		
BP Classification	SBP (mm Hg)	DBP (mm Hg)
Normal	<120	<80
Prehypertension	120–139	80–89
Stage 1 hypertension	140–159	90–99
Stage 2 hypertension	≥160	≥100

Abbreviations: BP, blood pressure; DBP, diastolic blood pressure; SBP, systolic blood pressure.
   Data from Chobanian AV, Bakris GL, Black HR, et al. Seventh report of the Joint National Committee on Prevention, Detection, Evaluation, and Treatment of High Blood Pressure. Hypertension 2003;42(6):1206–52.

cases that were cancelled because of presentation of severe hypertension did not result in normalization of blood pressure when the procedure was rescheduled.

For stage 3 hypertension (systolic blood pressure >180 mm Hg and diastolic blood pressure >110 mm Hg), the potential benefits of delaying surgery to optimize the effects of antihypertensive medications should be weighed against the risk of delaying the procedure. Most anesthesia practitioners delay surgery for patients with diastolic blood pressure more than 110 mm Hg, because these patients are thought to be at increased risk of perioperative dysrhythmias, myocardial ischemia, infarction, or stroke. However, a randomized trial by Weksler and colleagues[8] was unable to show a benefit to delaying surgery.

The goal for hypertensive patients is to maintain a stable, smooth intraoperative course. Despite adequate blood pressure control on a routine basis, patients with a history of hypertension on antihypertensive medication are still prone to increases in blood pressure intraoperatively. β-Blockers and calcium channel blockers should be continued on the day of surgery. Tachycardia, hypertension, angina, and MI can occur when β-blockers and calcium channel blockers are abruptly discontinued.[4] It may be optimal to hold angiotensin-converting enzyme (ACE) inhibitors and angiotensin receptor blockers (ARBs) for 24 to 48 hours preoperatively because of their association with increased intraoperative hypotension. This requirement should be determined on a case-by-case basis. Patients undergoing procedures with a high risk of hypovolemia and hypotension should have ACE inhibitors and ARBs held preoperatively.

Perioperative hypertension often occurs during the induction of anesthesia. It also presents intraoperatively associated with acute pain-induced sympathetic stimulation (**Table 2**). Postoperative hypertension can be associated with pain, hypothermia, hypoxia, or intravascular volume overload. The acute discontinuation of antihypertensive medication (withdrawal syndrome) also results in perioperative hypertension.[9]

Perioperative hypertension can contribute to:
- Increased risk of stroke
- Renal dysfunction
- Surgical bleeding
- Triggering of hyperinflammatory and procoagulant conditions
- Exacerbation of ischemic mitral regurgitation
- Acute pulmonary edema in the elderly

Table 2	
Causes of intraoperative hypertension	
Related to preexisting disease	Chronic hypertension, increased intracranial pressure, autonomic hyperreflexia, aortic dissection, early acute MI
Related to surgery	Prolonged tourniquet time, after cardiopulmonary bypass, aortic cross-clamping, after carotid endarterectomy
Related to anesthetic	Pain, inadequate depth of anesthesia, catecholamine release, malignant hyperthermia, shivering, hypoxia, hypercarbia, hypothermia, hypervolemia, blood pressure cuff too small, intra-arterial transducer positioned too low
Related to medication	Rebound hypertension (from acute discontinuation of clonidine, β-blockers, or methyldopa), systemic absorption of vasoconstrictors (local with epinephrine), intravenous dye (indigo carmine)
Other	Bladder distension, hypoglycemia

Adapted from Duke J. Blood pressure disturbances. In: Duke J, editor. Anesthesia Secrets. 4th edition. Philadelphia: Elsevier; 2011. p. 201–6.

- Increases in myocardial oxygen consumption and left ventricular end-diastolic pressure contributing to subendocardial low perfusion and myocardial ischemia[6]

Considerations:

- Hypertensive patients tend to have an exaggerated response to laryngoscopy and intubation, hence a fine balance of anesthetic agents, narcotics, and β-blockers helps to blunt this sympathetic response.
- Hypertensive patients are hypovolemic. Chronic vasoconstriction results in volume contraction and a greater susceptibility to hypotension from the vasodilating and cardiac-depressant effects of anesthetics.[4]
- It is ideal to maintain blood pressure within 20% of the patient's baseline mean pressure.
- It is critical for practitioners to remain vigilant in anticipating intraoperative events (eg, deepening the patient with anesthetics and narcotics to prevent an exaggerated sympathetic response to incision).
- Hypotension should be immediately treated by decreasing volatile agents, fluid administration, or vasopressors to maintain blood pressure within 20% of the patient's baseline.
- Emergence from anesthesia can also be correlated with hypertensive responses and is a time to titrate more narcotic and intravenous antihypertensive medications to continue a smooth course to the recovery area. **Table 3** reviews intraoperative antihypertensives.

MYOCARDIAL INFARCTION/ISCHEMIA

Perioperative MI (PMI) is an important predictor of morbidity and mortality following noncardiac surgery.[10] It has been reported that 8% of all patients undergoing surgery show evidence of significant myocardial injury.[11] Therefore, prevention of PMI is vital to improving postoperative outcomes. The preoperative assessment of cardiac risk, precise evaluation intraoperatively, and close assessment postoperatively involve multidisciplinary staff to appropriately monitor, recognize, and implement prompt treatment.

The most recent universal definition of MI is based on the increase or decrease in levels of cardiac biomarkers (specifically troponin) in the setting of myocardial ischemia: cardiac symptoms, electrocardiogram (ECG) changes (ST changes, new left bundle branch block, or development of Q waves), or imaging findings.[12] In one study, most ischemic events (67%) started at the end of surgery and emergence

| Table 3 | | | |
| Antihypertensive medications | | | |
Drug	Dose	Onset	Duration
Nitroprusside	0.5–10 μg/kg/min	30–60 s	1–5 min
Nitroglycerin	0.5–10 μg/kg/min	1 min	3–5 min
Esmolol	0.5 mg/kg over 1 min	1 min	12–20 min
Labetalol	5–20 mg	1–2 min	4–8 h
Hydralazine	5–20 mg	5–20 min	4–8 h
Nifedipine (sublingual)	10 mg	5–10 min	4 h
Nicardipine	0.25–0.5 mg or 5–15 mg/h	1–5 min	3–4 h

Data from Morgan GE, Mikhail MS, Murray MJ. Anesthesia for patients with cardiovascular disease. Clinical Anesthesiology. 4th edition. New York: McGraw-Hill; 2006. p. 451.

from anesthesia.[13] This period of time is characterized by an increase in heart rate, blood pressure, and sympathetic stimulation. Increases in arterial blood pressure, heart rate, and cardiac contractility lead to subendocardial ischemia by increasing myocardial oxygen demands in the presence of underlying CAD.[10] An MI occurs when oxygen supply is inadequate to meet myocardial demand. The procoagulant and antifibrinolytic activity induced by surgery can trigger coronary artery thrombosis in underlying CAD.[10]

Two separate mechanisms can lead to PMI[12]:

- Acute coronary syndrome (type 1 PMI)
- Prolonged myocardial oxygen supply demand imbalance (type 2 PMI) in the presence of stable CAD

ACUTE CORONARY SYNDROME (TYPE 1 PERIOPERATIVE MYOCARDIAL INFARCTION)

Acute coronary syndrome occurs when plaque undergoes spontaneous rupture or erosion, leading to coronary thrombosis, ischemia, and infarction.[10] Rupture is most common during strenuous physical activity or emotional stress. Stressors that are common to the perioperative setting can contribute and include physiologic and emotional stresses, and increased postoperative procoagulants. Activation of the sympathetic nervous system increases the concentration of catecholamines leading to tachycardia and hypertension, which can exert shear stress resulting in rupture of the plaques. The combination of increased prothrombotic and reduced fibrinolytic activity could initiate propagation and total occlusion of a coronary artery.[1]

MYOCARDIAL OXYGEN SUPPLY-DEMAND IMBALANCE (TYPE 2 PERIOPERATIVE MYOCARDIAL INFARCTION)

Tachycardia is the most common cause of type 2 PMI. Heart rates greater than 80 or 90 beats per minute (bpm) in patients with significant CAD who have preoperative resting heart rates of 50 to 60 bpm can lead to ischemia and PMI, showing a low threshold for ischemia after surgery.[1] Postoperative hypotension, hypertension, anemia, hypoxemia, and hypercarbia all aggravate ischemia.

Most (>80%) PMIs are asymptomatic, of the non–Q-wave type, and are commonly preceded by ST segment depression rather than elevation.[10] The cause of perioperative MI is highly debated between a supply-demand mismatch and plaque rupture. The following common findings in PMI cases have led to the opinion that prolonged stress-induced myocardial ischemia is the likely primary cause of PMI[10]:

- Increases in heart rate preceding the ischemic episodes
- ST segment depression rather than elevation during episodes
- Non–Q-wave rather than Q-wave MIs in almost all cases
- Lack of visible thrombus or ruptured plaque in patients who underwent coronary angiography following PMI

MIs are classified according to their location, as shown in **Table 4**.

PREVENTION

Practitioners are encouraged to identify patients' cardiac risks preoperatively using 6 independent predictors of major cardiac complications that have been highlighted in the Lee Revised Cardiac Risk Index. These predictors are high-risk surgery, ischemic heart disease, congestive heart failure, cerebrovascular disease, preoperative

Table 4
Classifications of MIs

Classification of MI	Layers Affected	ECG Changes
Transmural/Q wave MI	Full thickness. Involves all 3 cardiac layers: the endocardium, myocardium, and epicardium	Changes in myocardial depolarization and repolarization: present as new Q waves, and ST segment elevation
Nontransmural/ non–Q wave/ subendocardial MI	Infarction and necrosis are not full thickness	Some of the muscle in the area can still depolarize and ST elevation may not occur; less likely to develop Q waves

Adapted from Urden LD, Stacy KM, Lough ME. Thelan's critical care nursing. 5th edition. St Louis (MO): Elsevier; 2006.

insulin-dependent diabetes mellitus, and preoperative serum creatinine level greater than 2.0 mg/dL.[14] The presence of 1 or more of these risk factors increases the incidence of postoperative cardiac complications such as death, cardiac arrest, complete heart block, acute MI, and pulmonary edema. B-adrenoreceptor blockers should be administered to patients with 1 or more factors that are known to be associated with a higher perioperative cardiac risk.[15] Although perioperative β-blockers have been proved to decrease the risk of MI, this benefit is accompanied by an increased risk of stroke, hypotension, and bradycardia postoperatively. Practitioners must remain vigilant to titrating dose to effect. Patients already on β-blockers should be maintained on them throughout the perioperative period for optimal outcomes.[11] In addition, 3-hydroxy-3-methylglutaryl-coenzyme A (HMG-CoA) reductase inhibitors should be continued perioperatively because abrupt withdrawal may cause plaque destabilization (**Box 1**).[16]

Dual Antiplatelet Therapy

- Current recommendations support dual antiplatelet therapy (usually clopidogrel and aspirin) for at least 4 weeks after bare metal stent placement and for at least a year after drug-eluting stent placement. Elective surgery during this period is discouraged.[1]
- If discontinuation of clopidogrel is necessary, continuing aspirin and restarting clopidogrel as soon as possible after surgery is recommended.[1]

Perioperative Management

- Increase fraction of inspired oxygen to 100%.
- Control heart rate with β-blockers.

Box 1
HMG-CoA reductase inhibitors (statins)

Atorvastatin

Lovastatin

Simvastatin

Fluvastatin

Rosuvastatin

Pravastatin

- It is imperative for practitioners to maintain a fine balance between myocardial oxygen supply and demand. All causes of tachycardia, hypertension, hypotension, anemia, and pain should be treated aggressively.[1]
- Maintain a low threshold for transfusion in patients with CAD. In the Perioperative Ischemic Evaluation (POISE) trial, bleeding (requiring >2 units of blood) and an increase in every 10 beats in baseline heart rate were significant predictors of perioperative MI.[17]
- Troponin is the gold standard in the diagnosis of acute coronary syndrome because of greater specificity and sensitivity; creatine kinase MB (CKMB) is less sensitive.
- After surgery, because of the influence of anesthesia and analgesic agents, symptoms of MI can be atypical or absent. Any patient with suggestive symptoms of MI should have a 12-lead ECG and serial troponin measurements.[2]

ARRHYTHMIAS

Perioperative arrhythmias are a common complication of surgery, particularly in the elderly population. The incidence of postoperative arrhythmia after cardiothoracic surgery ranges from 30% to 40%, and it ranges from 4% to 20% for noncardiac surgeries.[18] The goal of intraoperative arrhythmia treatment is to treat immediate hemodynamic problems and prevent progression of serious arrhythmias. The first step in managing an arrhythmia depends on the hemodynamic effects of the rhythm.

Bradyarrhythmias are most often related to the fluctuation of vagal tone caused by direct surgical injury or local edema.[18] It is important to evaluate whether the decrease in heart rate is affecting perfusion. If the arrhythmia is associated with loss of atrial synchronous contraction then it can decrease cardiac output, especially in elderly patients. This decrease would lead to hypotension, decreased coronary perfusion pressure, and myocardial ischemia. Symptomatic bradycardia can be treated with ephedrine, atropine, or glycopyrrolate. In patients unresponsive to these intravenous medications, refer to the advanced cardiac life support guidelines for pacing.

Atrial fibrillation is the most common type of sustained supraventricular tachycardia, particularly in the elderly. Common factors that may contribute to perioperative atrial fibrillation include[18]:

- Increased sympathetic activation
- Blood loss
- Fluid shifts
- β-Blocker withdrawal
- Hypoglycemia or hyperglycemia
- Electrolyte disturbances

See **Table 5** for arrhythmias and their management.

AUTONOMIC DYSREFLEXIA

Autonomic dysreflexia (AD) is a medical emergency that can occur in patients with spinal cord injuries (SCIs) at or above the T6 level. The reflex response is initiated by cutaneous or visceral stimulation (not necessarily noxious) below the level of the spinal cord transection.[19] This sensation commonly originates in the bowel or bladder and enters the spinal cord via intact peripheral nerves (denoted by the letter A in **Fig. 1**). This input travels up the spinal cord, resulting in a reflex sympathetic discharge from the thoracolumbar sympathetic nerves (B). Intense vasoconstriction and

Table 5
Arrhythmias and management

Cardiac Dysrhythmia	Signs	Treatment	Management
Paroxysmal supraventricular tachycardia	Heart rate 160–180 bpm initiated by tissue above the AV node	Hemodynamically unstable: synchronized cardioversion (50–100 J) Hemodynamically stable: attempt vagal maneuvers Pharmacologic treatment: adenosine (6 mg, 12 mg, 12 mg), calcium channel blockers (verapamil, diltiazem), β-blockers	Avoid factors contributing to ectopy such as increased sympathetic tone, electrolyte imbalances, and acid-base alterations
Atrial flutter	Organized atrial rhythm with rate 250–350 bpm and varying degrees of AV block Atrial rate/ventricular rate is usually 2:1	Hemodynamically unstable: cardioversion (50–100 J) Hemodynamically stable: patients in flutter >48 h should be anticoagulated Pharmacologic treatment: amiodarone, diltiazem, or verapamil. The goal is to control the ventricular rate (none of these drugs is likely to convert flutter to sinus rhythm)	If flutter occurs before induction of anesthesia, surgery should be postponed If flutter occurs during procedure, follow treatment guidelines
Atrial fibrillation	Loss of coordinated atrial contractions and rapid ventricular rates Multiple areas of the atria depolarize and contract in a disorganized fashion (quivering)	Hemodynamically unstable: synchronized cardioversion (100–200 J) Hemodynamically stable: rate control Pharmacologic treatment to achieve rate control: amiodarone (150 mg IV over 10 min, then 1 mg/min for 6 h, then 0.5 mg/min for 18 h), propafenone, ibutilide, sotalol, β-blockers, calcium channel blockers, digoxin (0.125–0.25 µg IV)	If new onset of atrial fibrillation before induction, surgery should be postponed Cardioversion if patient is unstable, or IV medications as vital signs allow Patients with chronic atrial fibrillation should be maintained on antidysrhythmic drugs perioperatively Maintain normal electrolytes Consider anticoagulation

VT	More than 3 consecutive ventricular premature beats or PVCs Heart rate >120 bpm Wide QRS (>0.12 s) No P waves	Pulseless VT: Follow ACLS algorithm Hemodynamically unstable VT with a pulse: synchronized cardioversion (100 J) Hemodynamically stable VT with a pulse: amiodarone 150 mg IV bolus followed by infusion 1 mg/min, sotalol 1.5 mg/kg IV, lidocaine 0.5–0.75 mg/kg IV, procainamide 20–50 mg/min IV	Investigate causes (Hs and Ts[a]) because this can become sustained or worsen into ventricular fibrillation Other causes: myocardial ischemia, PVC landing on a T-wave, drug toxicity, or electrolyte imbalances
Ventricular fibrillation	Irregular ventricular rhythm resulting in no cardiac output	AHA advanced cardiac life support algorithm 200-J biphasic defibrillation (repeat every 2 min with shockable rhythm) CPR 30:2 for 2 min following shock (no pause to check rhythm or pulse) Epinephrine every 3–5 min Amiodarone 300 mg IV bolus (first dose), 150 mg IV (second dose)	Consider possible causes (Hs and Ts[a])

Abbreviations: ACLS, advanced cardiac life support; AV, atrioventricular; CPR, cardiopulmonary resuscitation; IV, intravenous; PVC, premature ventricular contractions; VT, ventricular tachycardia.

[a] The Hs and Ts are hypovolemia, hypoxia, hydrogen ion (acidosis), hypokalemia/hyperkalemia, hypothermia, tension pneumothorax, tamponade, toxins, and thrombosis (coronary or pulmonary).

Data from Neumar RW, Otto CW, Link MS, et al. Part 8: adult advanced cardiovascular life support: 2010 American Heart Association guidelines for cardiopulmonary resuscitation and emergency cardiovascular care. Circulation 2010;122(18 Suppl 3):S729–67. http://dx.doi.org/10.1161/circulationaha.110.970988.

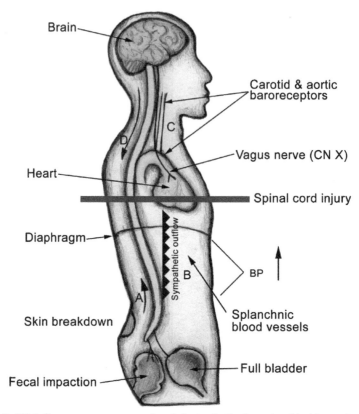

Fig. 1. AD. (A) Reflex response commonly originates in the bowel or bladder and enters the spinal cord via intact peripheral nerves. (B) This input travels up the spinal cord resulting in a reflex sympathetic discharge from the thoracolumbar sympathetic nerves. (C) Intense vasoconstriction and hypertension occur. The brain detects this hypertension through intact carotid and aortic baroreceptors in the neck. (D) The brain attempts to minimize the hypertensive response via two pathways. First, the brain attempts to send inhibitory impulses, however, these are unable to travel to the sympathetic outflow levels because of the cord injury. Secondly, the brain attempts to lower blood pressure by slowing the heart rate via the vagus nerve, therefore, bradycardia ensues yet hypertension persists. bp, blood pressure; CN X, Cranial Nerve X, Vagus Nerve. (Image reprinted with permission from Medscape Reference (http://emedicine.medscape.com/), 2014. Available at: http://emedicine.medscape.com/article/322809-overview.)

hypertension occur. The brain detects this hypertension through intact carotid and aortic baroreceptors in the neck (C). The brain attempts to inhibit the sympathetic discharge, but these impulses are blocked by the SCI. In addition, the brain attempts to reduce blood pressure by slowing the heart rate via the vagus nerve. This compensatory bradycardia is inadequate and hypertension continues. The sympathetics prevail below the injury and the parasympathetics prevail above the injury.

Despite the loss of sensation below the level of the injury, it is important to recognize that surgical procedures can still cause AD.[20] Up to 90% of individuals with cord injury undergoing surgery with topical anesthesia or no anesthesia develop AD.[20] Case reports of AD highlight that it can occur intraoperatively and postoperatively. Special attention should be directed to postoperative patients at risk for AD in the recovery area because the effects of anesthetic drugs are wearing off.

Assessment

AD is characterized by intense vasoconstriction below the site of the lesion and cutaneous vasodilation above the site of the lesion. Acute increase of blood pressure is the most common presenting sign, leading to severe hypertension and bradycardia (baroreceptor reflex).

Untreated AD can progress to seizures, intracranial hemorrhage, or MI.

An increase in systolic blood pressure greater than 20 to 30 mm Hg is considered a dysreflexic episode.[20] It is critical to keep in mind that resting blood pressure in patients with high cervical or thoracic injuries may be lower than normal, and therefore an AD episode can present with what seems to be a healthy or slightly increased blood pressure.

Management

Initial treatment involves placing the patient in the upright position to take advantage of any orthostatic reduction in blood pressure and loosening any tight clothing or constrictive devices.[20] Search for and eliminate the stimulus, which is bowel or bladder in 85% of cases.[20] Deepen anesthesia for vasodilatory effects and administer direct-acting vasodilators such as nifedipine or nitrates (**Table 6**).

CARDIAC TAMPONADE

Cardiac tamponade is the accumulation of blood in the pericardial sac. The pericardial sac normally contains up to 50 mL of serous fluid.[21] The accumulation of blood that occurs with tamponade results in external pressure that compresses the atria and ventricles and therefore impairs filling. Cardiac preload, cardiac output, and blood pressure are all strongly affected. Because stroke volume becomes fixed, cardiac output becomes dependent on heart rate and the sympathetic system is activated as a reflex. There are many reasons for development of pericardial effusions, with few progressing to tamponade. The gradual accumulation of pericardial fluid allows time for compensation and may not result in severe presentation of tamponade. The most common causes of large pericardial effusions requiring pericardial window

Table 6 Direct-acting vasodilators			
Drug	Class	Mechanism	Dose
Nifedipine (Adalat, Procardia)	Calcium channel blocker	↓ Peripheral vascular resistance, ↓ systolic and diastolic	In general given for acute episode of AD, 10 mg. Bite and swallow
Nitrates (nitroglycerine, Nitrostat, Nitro-Bid)	Nitrates	Relaxation of vascular smooth muscle, peripheral arteries, and veins	0.5–10 µg/kg/min IV titrated to effect
Captopril	ACE inhibitor	Specific competitive inhibitor of ACE	25 mg sublingually

Data from Krassioukov A, Warburton DE, Teasell R, et al. Spinal cord rehabilitation evidence research team. A systematic review of the management of autonomic dysreflexia after spinal cord injury. Arch Phys Med Rehabil 2009;90(4):682–95.

surgery include effusions associated with malignancy or end-stage renal disease, those occurring after cardiac surgery, and idiopathic effusions. Acute tamponade can develop from direct chest trauma, ruptured aortic aneurysms, and effusions secondary to percutaneous cardiac interventions (such as catheter ablations for atrial fibrillation, pacemaker lead changes).

Treatment of acute pericardial tamponade requires immediate drainage, usually by needle pericardiocentesis using echocardiographic or fluoroscopic guidance.[21] Removal of small amounts of pericardial fluid can improve hemodynamics. Surgical drainage can also be accomplished via pericardial window formation, a small anterior thoracotomy, or formation of a pericardial-peritoneal window.[21]

Clinical Findings

- Tachycardia
- Dyspnea
- Pulsus paradoxus (exaggerated decrease in systolic blood pressure >10 mm Hg during inspiration)
- Beck triad: increased central venous pressure with neck vein distension, muffled heart sounds, and hypotension
- Pulseless electrical activity in the absence of hypovolemia and tension pneumothorax suggests cardiac tamponade

Management

Immediate treatment is required to remove the fluid from the pericardial space. Management is designed to maintain the stroke volume until the pericardial sac is open (this may involve administration of fluids to increase preload). Patients with tamponade are at risk of severe hypotension and cardiac arrest with anesthesia induction. For this reason, numerous case reports have concluded that pericardial drainage can be accomplished with local anesthetic infiltration.[21] Sedative/analgesics can be used as needed (ketamine, midazolam, or fentanyl). As an alternative, initial drainage can be accomplished with local anesthetic infiltration, and, after hemodynamics have improved, general anesthesia can be induced.[21] Data suggest that despite brief vasopressor requirements following induction of general anesthesia, there is no difference in outcomes between general and local anesthesia.[21] If general anesthesia is decided, those anesthetics that minimally depress cardiac function and limit vasodilation are warranted (opt for ketamine or etomidate).

Positive pressure ventilation can increase vascular resistance and decrease right ventricular outflow, further exacerbating left septal shift, impairing left ventricle filling, and worsening hypotension. For this reason, maintenance of spontaneous ventilation is recommended. If general anesthesia is necessary, avoiding large tidal volumes and high peak airway pressures minimizes the impact of ventilation on hemodynamics.[21]

TENSION PNEUMOTHORAX

Tension pneumothorax is a rare intraoperative event, occurring most often in emergency department or intensive care settings. Tension pneumothorax occurs when air accumulates within the pleural cavity. When this pressure becomes too great, the mediastinum shifts to the opposite hemithorax and causes compression on the contralateral lung and blood vessels. The hallmark signs are hypotension,

Box 2
Causes of tension pneumothorax
Migration of laparoscopic gas (CO_2 under pressure can pass from abdominal cavity into pleura)
Direct pulmonary barotrauma
Central line insertion
Brachial plexus blockade
Thoracic epidural placement
Use of an airway exchange catheter
Traumatic intubation
Jet ventilation

hypoxemia, tachycardia, increased central venous pressure, and increased airway pressure.[22]

During surgery, tension pneumothorax has occurred as a result of the causes listed in **Box 2**.[23]

Assessment

- Sudden decrease in pulmonary compliance
- Increase in airway pressure
- Increase in end tidal pressure of carbon dioxide and $Paco_2$
- Unchanged or decreased Pao_2
- Unchanged or decreased blood pressure
- Absent breath sounds on affected side
- Asymmetric chest wall movement
- Tracheal shift

Management

Immediate treatment is crucial. A fiberoptic bronchoscopy may initially be completed to rule out endobronchial intubation. The chest can be decompressed with insertion of 16-gauge or 18-gauge catheter into the second or third interspace anteriorly or the fourth or fifth interspace laterally. A rush of air is heard when decompression occurs.

SUMMARY

Despite thorough preoperative evaluation and assessment of cardiac risk, cardiac emergencies still occur. To optimize patient outcomes, perioperative providers must remain alert for changes in patient status and familiar with the recommended management of these emergencies. Patients with hypertension, CAD, and history of arrhythmias must be optimized on medication regimens before elective and nonemergent procedures. Cardiac emergencies such as MI, tamponade, and AD should be recognized quickly and treated promptly.

REFERENCES

1. Landesberg G, Beattie S, Mosseri M, et al. Perioperative myocardial infarction. Circulation 2009;119(22):2936–44.

2. Shammash JB, Kimmel SE. Perioperative myocardial infarction after noncardiac surgery. In: Solomon S, Mohler ER, Bax JJ, et al, editors. UpToDate. Waltham, MA: UpToDate; 2014.

3. Gillespie CD, Hurvitz KA, Centers for Disease Control and Prevention. Prevalence of hypertension and controlled hypertension: United States 2007–2010. MMWR Surveill Summ 2013;62(3):144–8.

4. Elisha S. Cardiovascular anatomy, physiology, pathophysiology, and anesthesia management. In: Nagelhout JJ, Plaus KL, editors. Nurse anesthesia. 4th edition. St Louis (MO): Saunders Elsevier; 2010. p. 487–90.

5. Chobanian AV, Bakris GL, Black HR, et al. Seventh report of the Joint National Committee on Prevention, Detection, Evaluation, and Treatment of High Blood Pressure. Hypertension 2003;42(6):1206–52.

6. Aronson S. Perioperative hypertensive emergencies. Curr Hypertens Rep 2014; 16(7):448.

7. Wax DB, Porter SB, Lin HM, et al. Association of preanesthesia hypertension with adverse outcomes. J Cardiothorac Vasc Anesth 2010;24(6):927–30.

8. Weksler N, Klein M, Szendro G, et al. The dilemma of immediate preoperative hypertension: to treat and operate, or to postpone surgery? J Clin Anesth 2003;15(3):179–83.

9. Varon J, Marik PE. Perioperative hypertension management. Vasc Health Risk Manag 2008;4(3):615–27.

10. Priebe HJ. Perioperative myocardial infarction: aetiology and prevention. Br J Anaesth 2005;95(1):3–19.

11. Wijeysundera DN, Duncan D, Nkonde-Price C, et al. Perioperative beta blockade in noncardiac surgery: a systemic review for the 2014 ACC/AHA guidelines on perioperative cardiovascular evaluation and management of patients undergoing noncardiac surgery guidelines. J Am Coll Cardiol 2014. http://dx.doi.org/10.1016/j.jacc.2014.07.939.

12. Thygesen K, Alpert JS, White HD. Universal definition of myocardial infarction. Eur Heart J 2007;28(20):2525–38.

13. Landesberg G, Mosseri M, Zahger D, et al. Myocardial infarction after vascular surgery: the role of prolonged, stress-induced, ST depression-type ischemia. J Am Coll Cardiol 2001;37(7):1839–45.

14. Lee TH, Marcantonio ER, Mangione CM, et al. Derivation and prospective validation of a simple index for prediction of cardiac risk of major noncardiac surgery. Circulation 1999;100(10):1043–9.

15. Kertai MD, Bax JJ, Klein J, et al. Is there any reason to withhold beta blockers from high-risk patients with coronary artery disease during surgery? Anesthesiology 2004;100(1):4–7.

16. Le Manach Y, Godet G, Coriat P, et al. The impact of postoperative discontinuation or continuation of chronic statin therapy on cardiac outcome after major vascular surgery. Anesth Analg 2007;104(6):1326–33.

17. POISE Study Group, Devereaux PJ, Yang H, et al. Effects of extended-release metoprolol succinate in patients undergoing non-cardiac surgery (POISE trial): a randomized controlled trial. Lancet 2008;371(9627):1839–47.

18. Melduni RM, Koshino Y, Shen WK. Management of arrhythmias in the perioperative setting. Clin Geriatr Med 2012;28(4):729–43.

19. Pasternak JJ, Lanier WL. Spinal cord disorders. In: Hines RL, Marschall KE, editors. Stoelting's anesthesia and co-existing disease. 5th edition. Philadelphia: Churchill Livingstone; 2008. p. 242–3.

20. Krassioukov A, Warburton DE, Teasell R, et al, Spinal Cord Rehabilitation Evidence Research Team. A systematic review of the management of autonomic dysreflexia after spinal cord injury. Arch Phys Med Rehabil 2009; 90(4):682–95.
21. O'Connor CJ, Tuman KJ. The intraoperative management of patients with pericardial tamponade. Anesthesiol Clin 2010;28(1):87–96.
22. Rieker M. Respiratory anatomy, physiology, pathophysiology, and anesthesia management. In: Nagelhout JJ, Plaus KL, editors. Nurse anesthesia. 4th edition. St Louis (MO): Saunders Elsevier; 2010. p. 618–9.
23. Finlayson GN, Chiang AB, Brodsky JB, et al. Intraoperative contralateral tension pneumothorax during pneumonectomy. Anesth Analg 2008;106(1):58–60.

Critical Care Nursing in Acute Postoperative Neurosurgical Patients

Christin Brooks, CRNA, MSNA, APRN

KEYWORDS

- Neurological • Postoperative • Neurosurgery • Craniotomy • Endovascular
- Intensive care

KEY POINTS

- Most postoperative neurologic patients, regardless of the disease process, face common risks and complications that require continuous monitoring to improve patient outcomes.
- Postoperative neurosurgical patients require an understanding of the unique needs that must be met by both the anesthesia and nursing staff.
- Surgical and endovascular neurologic patients require a high acuity of care. Mainstays of postoperative care include continuous assessment in areas of level of consciousness, hemodynamics, temperature, pain, seizures, nausea, and fluid therapy.

CONSIDERATIONS OF POSTNEUROSURGICAL PATIENTS REGARDLESS OF PATHOLOGIC CONDITION

Neurologic Assessment

Frequent and thorough neurologic assessments are paramount to rapid intervention in a deteriorating or worsening patient condition. Many facilities implement the use of hourly neurologic assessments through the routine use of the Glasgow Coma Scale (GCS) (**Table 1**).

The objectivity of the GCS allows for a standard measurement of a patient's neurologic status. Nurses can use this scale by assessing 3 components of a patient's condition via eye, motor, and verbal response. Deteriorations in a patient's GCS will require prompt nursing intervention and notification of the neurosurgical team. On admission of acute neurosurgical patients to the intensive care unit (ICU), it is imperative to perform a baseline neurologic examination. This baseline examination will allow the nurse to quickly detect any potential deterioration in the neurologic condition during patient care. This examination also allows for continuity of care in the transitional period from the postoperative period through the transfer of care to the ICU.

No disclosures.
Department of Anesthesiology, Yale-New Haven Hospital, 20 York Street, New Haven, CT 06510, USA
E-mail address: christin_brooks@hotmail.com

Crit Care Nurs Clin N Am 27 (2015) 33–45
http://dx.doi.org/10.1016/j.cnc.2014.10.002   ccnursing.theclinics.com

Table 1 Glasgow Coma Scale (GCS)		
Action	**Reaction**	**Value**
Eye opening	Spontaneously opens eyes	4
	Opens eyes to verbal stimulation	3
	Opens eyes to painful stimulation	2
	No response to stimulation	1
Verbal	Oriented	5
	Confused	4
	Inappropriate to questions	3
	Incomprehensible	2
	No response to stimulation	1
Motor	Follows commands	6
	Localizes extremities to pain	5
	Withdraws extremities to pain	4
	Decorticate movement	3
	Decerebrate movement	2
	No response to stimulation	1
Total	Normal neurologic examination	15
	Coma	8 or less
	Unresponsive	3

Adapted from Teasdale G, Jennett B. Assessment of coma and impaired consciousness: a practical scale. Lancet 1974;2:81, with permission; and Jennett B. Assessment of the severity of head injury. J Neurol Neurosurg Psychiatry 1976;39:647.

Another key element of the nursing neurologic assessment includes frequent monitoring of pupil appearance and reactivity, commonly known as PERRLA (pupils that are equally round and reactive to light and accommodation). Changes in pupil appearance or sluggish reactivity to light can be an indicator of a patient's worsening neurologic prognosis. The neurosurgical evaluation should also include the baseline and continued monitoring of all extremities' power and mobility to command. Any change in a patient's level of consciousness (LOC) or deviation from baseline assessment requires prompt notification to the medical care team.

Testing and Imaging

Routine tests for neurologic conditions include the use of a computerized tomography (CT) scan and MRI for more accurate diagnostic depictions of a patient's clinical picture. Initial imaging may occur in the emergency department on the patient's admission to the hospital. Subsequent testing is commonly used as a daily prognostic indicator or with a change in neurologic status that may require surgical or endovascular intervention. Diagnostic tests may need to be performed on critically ill patients who require mechanical ventilation. Nurses should anticipate that patients suffering from acute brain trauma or a diminished GCS may require mechanical ventilation while transported for testing. Mechanically ventilated patients must be closely monitored with emphasis on protecting the endotracheal tube (ETT). Transfer of these patients to procedural and testing areas within health care institutions may call for increased assistance, along with sedatives and portable ventilators to ensure patient safety. Patients requiring mechanical ventilation via an ETT also require a nurse who is skilled in critical care management.

Sedation of Critical Neurologic Patients

Pharmacologic measures may be required to sedate patients in order to tolerate mechanical ventilation. Pain control and the need to rest patients after a critical injury or surgery are additional indications for sedation. At times patients fail to meet the criteria for extubation and remain intubated following general anesthesia and neurosurgery. Typically short-acting sedatives and narcotics are preferred for sedation because of the importance of routine and hourly neurologic examinations. Commonly used sedatives include propofol, fentanyl, and midazolam. Long-acting drugs that obscure neurologic status can give false impressions of a worsening neurologic condition and should be avoided if possible. Ideally, postsurgical patients require a neurologic examination on emergence from anesthesia in order to assess for potential surgical complications and obtain a baseline. A thorough report from the anesthesia provider after general anesthesia will include all medications given in order to give the critical care team an accurate time frame for any lingering side effects. During the handoff between the anesthesia provider and the critical care team, it is recommended to review the baseline neurologic status of patients before surgery. Any deviations from either the presurgical or postsurgical baseline require prompt notification to the surgical and ICU team.

Intracranial Pressure

The intracranial space is considered a fixed space. This space is considered to be a fixed box containing the brain, blood, and cerebral spinal fluid (CSF). Intracranial pressure (ICP) is the pressure exerted on the brain, blood, and CSF within the cranial vault. In the healthy individual without neurologic disease, normal ICP values range between 5 and 15 mm Hg.[1]

In the brain, autoregulation ensures that adequate perfusion of cerebral blood flow (CBF) occurs regardless of variances in blood pressure. This response is ideal in the presence of either high or low arterial pressures, as it causes a compensatory dilation or constriction of arterial vasculature in response to overwhelming or inadequate blood pressures.[1] Cerebral perfusion pressure (CPP) relies on 2 variables, mean arterial pressure (MAP) and ICP.

$$MAP - ICP = CPP$$

This formula is used to calculate and assess the CPP to ensure adequate perfusion to integral brain tissue is occurring. Normal values for CPP are 50 to 150 mm Hg. At more and less than these values, cerebral ischemia or cerebral edema can occur as cerebral autoregulation is lost.

According to Forsyth and colleagues,[2] "Brain swelling accompanied by raised ICP resulted in inadequate cerebral perfusion with well oxygenated blood. Detection of raised ICP could be useful in alerting clinicians to the need to improve cerebral perfusion, with consequent reductions in brain injury."[2] Changes in CSF volume or structures can cause a compensatory increase in ICP because of the fixed space the brain lies within. Increases in ICP in conjunction with the inability to maintain CPP can present clinically as a deteriorating neurosurgical assessment that the nurse is constantly in watch for. In order to intervene or prevent associated complications of increased ICP, it is imperative to frequently evaluate and assess LOC.

ICP is commonly measured via an external ventricular drain (EVD) or ventriculostomy. Placement of this device by neurosurgeons can also allow for drainage of CSF from the ventricles of the brain in the presence of increased ICP. Direct measurement of increasing ICP is particularly beneficial in the care of patients in a comatose or chemically paralyzed state, whereby routine assessments are invalid.[2] The EVD is, therefore, not only a monitoring device but also a direct intervention for increased ICP.

Increased intracranial pressure: signs and symptoms

Signs and symptoms that the nursing team must be aware of include worsening of GCS score with coma, nausea, vomiting, headache, or papilledema.[1]

Without intervention, increasing ICP and inadequate CPP cannot only lead to cerebral ischemia and neurologic deficits but also, in severe cases, to cerebral herniation through the foramen magnum. Pressure on the brain and cranial nerves can lead to cardiorespiratory arrest and ultimately death. A phenomenon associated with greatly increased ICP, compromised CPP, and ultimately a sign of impending cerebral herniation is called the Cushing triad. The 3 physiologic signs and symptoms that characterize the Cushing triad include irregular breathing, bradycardia less than 50 beats per minute, and hypertension with a widening pulse pressure.

Common causes of increased ICP
- CSF outflow obstruction, jugular venous obstruction
- Cerebral edema/cerebral hemorrhage
- Tracheal stimulation (suctioning, coughing, bucking) increases ICP on average 15 mm Hg[3]
- Valsalva maneuver and positive end-expiratory pressure greater than 20 cm H_2O[4]

Interventions to decrease elevated intracranial pressure

It is important to treat increased ICP promptly, as values exceeding 20 mm Hg require immediate intervention.[1] Commonly used nursing interventions to quickly achieve a reduction in ICP are listed in **Table 2**.

Table 2
Nursing interventions to decrease elevated ICP

Nursing Intervention	Mechanism of Action
Elevating head of bed >30°	Allows for venous drainage
Hyperventilation, rapidly decreases ICP	Effective only for 6–12 h by decreasing CO_2 concentrations in blood causing vasoconstriction of cerebral vessels[1]
Drain CSF from EVD or lumbar drain	Immediately decreases volume of CSF
Infusion of hyperosmotic drugs Mannitol: 0.25–0.5 g/kg IV over 15–30 min	Osmotic diuresis of brain, lowers ICP and increases urine output, may cause rebound increased ICP[5]
Furosemide	0.1–2.0 mg/kg IV decreases sodium transport in brain[4]
Corticosteroids: dexamethasone, prednisone	Decreases ICP in patients with vasogenic edema caused by brain tumors[6]
Barbiturates, propofol, benzodiazepines	Sedative effects particularly useful in acute brain trauma, decreasing brain activity and decreasing CMRO2 requirements[4]
Maintenance of normal blood glucose	Osmotic shifts causing increased ICP[7]

Abbreviations: CMRO2, cerebral metabolic rate of oxygen consumption; CO_2, carbon dioxide; IV, intravenous.
Data from Refs.[1,4–7]

NURSING CONSIDERATIONS AFTER CRANIOTOMY/CRANIECTOMY

Following neurosurgical procedures, nursing staff should closely monitor for signs and symptoms of pain, anxiety, and changes in LOC by monitoring vital signs and physical assessment. As demonstrated earlier, these circumstances can cause an increase in ICP and cause additional brain injury. Hemorrhage is an immediate postoperative concern, and a thorough assessment can help to identify this complication. Intraoperatively, a piece of bone from the skull is removed to gain surgical access to brain tissue. Because of the nature of the surgery, this bone flap will either be replaced (craniotomy) or removed temporarily (craniectomy) at the conclusion of the procedure. After a craniectomy, this bone flap will be removed temporarily to allow for cerebral tissue swelling. Bulging of the bone flap site will be noticeable if intracranial hypertension is allowed to persist. Peak cerebral edema often occurs 48 to 72 hours postoperatively. The surgical site must be closely protected and monitored for signs and symptoms of infection and wound compromise.[4]

Patients having undergone craniotomy or craniectomy are at risk for hemorrhage, intracranial hematoma, and cerebral edema in the immediate postoperative period. There are many factors that cause an increased risk for complications in neurologic patients. These common complications pertaining to all postoperative neurologic patients are focused on in the following sections.

Emergence from General Anesthesia

Sympathetic stimulation on emergence from general anesthesia, endotracheal stimulation via mechanical ventilation, and stimulation from the surgical site can all result in a catecholamine increase. The catecholamine increase presents as tachycardia and arterial hypertension, which are factors that contribute to the risk of hemorrhage. Patients who are extubated early in the operating room may demonstrate a decreased sympathetic surge compared with patients who have a delayed emergence from anesthesia and are extubated in the ICU.[3,8] Early emergence from anesthesia will facilitate the identification of potential complications by creating ideal conditions to perform an early neurologic assessment. Prompt recognition of complications postoperatively will decrease or limit damage to brain tissue.

Hemodynamic and respiratory stability must be present in order to safely discontinue mechanical ventilation. When a patient returns from the operating room intubated, there is direct stimulation from the endotracheal tube and mechanical ventilation. These factors increase cardiac response and metabolic stress; limiting exposure to these stressors may decrease complications.[3,8] If patients are unable to meet certain extubation criteria or are unstable hemodynamically, then early extubation after anesthesia may not be an option. Continued sedation to facilitate mechanical ventilation along with immediate admission to the ICU is the safest course of action for a patient who does not meet the extubation criteria postoperatively. In both situations, close monitoring of the hemodynamic status is imperative to prevent neurologic complications.

Nursing considerations
- Maintain a blood pressure of no more than 20% to 30% greater than the preoperative baseline because of the increased risk for intracranial hemorrhage and cerebral edema.[5]
- Nursing interventions to maintain normal blood pressure and heart rate can decrease the risk of complications. The surgeon or intensivist prescribes the goal parameters.

- To treat hypertension and tachycardia, the use of beta-blocking agents, such as labetalol and metoprolol, should be anticipated. Hydralazine is also commonly used.

Temperature

During neurosurgical procedures, it is common practice for anesthesia personnel to allow cooling of a patient's core temperature. Hypothermia (<36°C) causes a complex cascade of reactions that reduce cerebral metabolic activity, which in turn decreases oxygen consumption in brain tissue. The cerebral metabolic rate of oxygen consumption (CMRO2) is directly related to increases in ICP.[9] During neurosurgery, the brain is at risk of being exposed to periods of low CBF. Anesthetic goals, therefore, institute protective measures to decrease cerebral oxygen requirements as well as overall consumption.[9]

General endotracheal anesthesia (GETA) combined with intraoperative hypothermia contribute to the cause of shivering in emerging patients. Shivering in neurologic patients can cause up to a 400% increase in oxygen consumption. Normothermic, nonshivering patients exhibit fewer oxygen demands.[9] Even mild hypothermia causes a decrease in the metabolism of most drugs, and lasting effects of anesthetics can be observed.[3] Following surgery and anesthesia, rewarming measures are initiated. It should be of note that patients may require additional warming on admission to the ICU. Hyperthermia may indicate other critical events; regardless of the presence of infection, it is associated with poorer outcomes.[10]

Nursing considerations
- Methods of rewarming can include forced-air warming devices, warming blankets, increased room temperature, and warming of intravenous fluids.
- Neurologic assessments may be delayed as sedative effects of anesthetic agents may be prolonged in hypothermic patients.
- It should be emphasized that the care team must be alerted to the presence of persistent hypothermia or even mild hyperthermia in postneurosurgical patients.

Pain Control

Postoperatively, most intracranial surgeries are associated with low analgesic requirements.[11] There are multiple reasons for this, most of which can be attributed to the lack of pain receptors that innervate brain tissues.[11] Anesthesia personnel ideally administer short-acting narcotics/anxiolytics that allow for quick emergence from general anesthesia and neurologic assessment. However, patients having undergone frontal craniotomy were shown to have increasing needs for pain control.[11] Pain and emergence from general anesthesia can cause undesirable hemodynamic changes and increased CMRO2 in the brain.[3,8]

Hyperventilation and increased work of breathing caused by pain can alter levels of carbon dioxide, lowering amounts in the bloodstream ($Paco_2$) causing vasoconstriction of cerebral vessels. Contrarily, a decreased respiratory rate and apnea associated with narcotic administration can cause cerebral vasodilation as $Paco_2$ levels increase.[4] Much effort has gone into the production and institution of guidelines to objectively measure and treat pain, agitation, and delirium in the ICU.[12]

Nursing considerations
- Pain can increase ICP and lead to changes in CBF, metabolism, and hemodynamics.[3,8] Analgesia can decrease pain, agitation, and delirium associated with the emergence from anesthesia in the postoperative setting.

- Narcotics should be used judiciously, as over sedation of neurosurgical patients can present as a worsening neurologic status, requiring intervention.

Fluid Therapy and Electrolyte Imbalance

Maintenance of euvolemia should be the goal intraoperatively and postoperatively in neurosurgical patients.[1,4,5,13] During craniotomy, patients are exposed to the risk of bleeding that may require the administration of isotonic crystalloid solutions or blood and blood products to maintain CPP and hemodynamic stability. Isotonic solutions are the standard of care in fluid administration for neurosurgical patients. Fluids containing glucose should be avoided, as hyperglycemia is associated with poorer outcomes. In neurologic patients, glucose is metabolized quickly and leads to the presence of free water contributing to cerebral edema.[13]

Intraoperatively, surgeons may request anesthesia personnel to administer diuretics, such as mannitol and furosemide, to decrease cerebral edema and optimize surgical conditions. These medications can contribute to electrolyte imbalances, hypovolemia, and hypotension in the postoperative period.

The most common electrolyte imbalance affecting neurologic patients is the plasma level of sodium. The implementation of fluid restriction to treat hyponatremia has fallen out of favor in critical care.[7] Hypertonic solutions, such as 3% saline, to treat hyponatremia and/or cerebral edema are effective, however, with fluid replacement not fluid restriction.[4,5] Hypertonic saline (HS) may be more effective than mannitol in the treatment of cerebral edema, as rebound increased ICP is not present and CSF production may be reduced.[13] Hypernatremia is a cause for concern with the administration of HS, and serial laboratory values should be drawn to monitor serum sodium levels. Cerebral pontine myelinolysis is a potentially disastrous but less commonly occurring side effect of too rapidly correcting sodium imbalances with HS.[4] Replacement of vital fluids and electrolytes while optimizing goals for euvolemia decreases morbidity and mortality in neurologic patients.[13]

Nursing considerations
- Signs and symptoms of hypovolemia include poor skin turgor, dry mouth, thirst, confusion, odd behavior, low urine output, tachycardia, and hypotension.
- Consider that neurologic patients (particularly if sedated) may not present with typical symptoms, and confusion may be a hallmark of hypovolemia not necessarily a neurologic emergency.
- Document accurate accounts of intake and output.

Postoperative Nausea and Vomiting

Nausea and vomiting can be an early sign of increased ICP and worsening neurologic status. There is also a high incidence of postoperative nausea and vomiting (PONV) associated with neurosurgical cases.[14] In particular, certain neurosurgical procedures, such as cortical resection for epilepsy, acoustic neuroma surgery, and microvascular decompression of cranial nerves, are at an increased risk of PONV.[14] This increase risk may be caused by direct or indirect stimulation of the chemoreceptor trigger zone or the area postrema during surgery.[14] Stimulation of these areas may increase the incidence of nausea and vomiting, and vagal stimulation may also be a cofactor.[1,14] During and after anesthesia, patients routinely receive antiemetic medications, such as ondansetron.

Nursing considerations
- Because of the nature of craniotomy/craniectomy, nurses should be aware of the potentially increased need for antiemetic drugs.

- Concomitant use of antiseizure medications, as in epilepsy, causes an increase in liver metabolism. This increase may result in decreased efficacy of antiemetics by increasing their metabolism and elimination in the bloodstream. Therefore, medications, such as ondansetron, may need to be redosed.[14]

Seizures

Neurologic conditions that are in close proximity to or directly involve the cerebral cortex have a higher incidence of seizures. Seizures are most likely exhibited with disorders such as epilepsy, brain tumor (40% of patients), and acute brain injury (intracranial hemorrhage and aneurysmal subarachnoid hemorrhage [SAH; 20% of patients]).[15] These patient populations benefit from the prophylactic administration of antiepileptic drug (AED) administration, although arbitrary and widespread use of AEDs has fallen out of favor.[15] In the instance of traumatic brain injury and SAH, seizure activity is most likely within the first 24 hours of hospital admission and anticonvulsants should be administered. In a meta-analysis, it was found that the use of prophylactic AEDs for other neurosurgical pathologies was inconclusive and should be avoided.[15] Preoperatively, patients are assessed for either continuation or a need for initiation of AED prophylaxis during surgery. Many anesthetic agents can inhibit seizure activity, which can increase the risk of seizure on emergence from anesthesia. Postoperatively, patients' continued need for anticonvulsant therapy should be assessed by critical care teams and administered accordingly.

Older AEDs, such as phenytoin, phenobarbital, and valproic acid, have deleterious side-effect profiles that may worsen the neurologic condition and increase the incidence of adverse events. Newer studies suggest the use of levetiracetam as an alternative to prevent seizures and, therefore, mitigate these side effects.[1,4,15] During a seizure, increased CMRO2 causes a resultant increase in CBF and ICP, which can lead to cerebral ischemia.[4] In addition, seizure activity can result in a loss of consciousness. Without cessation of seizure activity there is a risk for cardiorespiratory compromise. Particularly of concern is the potential for airway compromise and loss of airway reflexes. Critical care nurses should be aware of the potential complications associated with seizures and seizure-prone patient populations.

Nursing considerations
- Maintain perioperative AED therapy, and discuss with anesthesia and surgical team about prophylaxis administration.
- The potential side-effect profile of AEDs can be lethal. Familiarize nursing staff with routes of administration, dosing, immediate side effects, and overall safety in the use of these medications (**Table 3**.)

Table 3
Seizure prophylaxis/treatment

Antiepileptic Drug	Dose
Phenytoin	Loading dose: 10–20 mg/kg IV at rate of no faster than 50 mg/min
Fosphenytoin	Loading dose: 15–20 mg/kg IV at rate of no faster than 100–150 mg/min
Phenobarbital	Loading dose: 6–8 mg/kg IV Maintenance dosage: 1–3 mg/kg/24 h IV

Abbreviation: IV, intravenous.
Data from Urden LD, Stacy KM, Lough ME. Thelan's critical care nursing diagnosis and management. 5th edition. St Louis (MO): Mosby; 2006.

- Immediate identification of seizure activity and supportive intervention include Advanced Cardiac Life Support (ACLS) with emphasis on airway, breathing, and circulation.
- Administer benzodiazepines (lorazepam most commonly used) for immediate cessation of seizurelike activity.

SPECIFIC CONSIDERATIONS IN ENDOVASCULAR SURGERY

There has become an increasing trend for patients with neurologic disease to undergo endovascular surgery.[16] Interventional radiologic (IR) procedures have shown a decrease in morbidity and mortality.[16] Patients can have endovascular procedures for a variety of reasons, but acute ischemic stroke (AIS) and SAH are the most common cases handled in IR. These endovascular interventions associated with these cases and resultant vasospasm are covered in the following sections. Nurses must continue a thorough assessment while maintaining constant communication with the surgical and ICU teams in the event of changes occurring in the patients' neurologic status. For this reason, it is recommended that nurses working in the IR suite possess critical care experience.

The neurologic patient population has unique needs that must be met while still focusing on the underlying neurologic process. Anesthetic management of endovascular patients varies greatly and can be administered as GETA or intravenous sedation. For patients with poor neurologic function, it may be safer to undergo GETA because of the disease process or to allow for complete immobility of patients during a meticulous and potentially dangerous procedure. Nursing staff must be aware that GETA may delay the neurologic examination and evaluation of cognitive function, especially when a patient does not meet the criteria for extubation at the end of the procedure.

Uniquely, critical care experience is also helpful in the IR suite, as procedures may be done with patient sedation administered by nurses. It is imperative that nurses are familiar with basic and advanced life support techniques should patients be unable to protect their airway at any time during the procedure, whether because of sedation or deteriorating neurologic status. An advantage of conscious sedation is that patients are able to interact with the surgical team and neurologic evaluation can take place simultaneously with the procedure. As with traditional neurosurgery before endovascular surgery or the administration of anesthetics/sedatives, baseline neurologic status must be evaluated and documented. Postoperatively, the patients' response to endovascular intervention and the potential for neurologic compromise require immediate evaluation of neurologic status.

Nursing considerations for all endovascular interventions

- Hemorrhage/hematoma formation postoperatively, most often femoral site
- Reversal of intraprocedural anticoagulation
- Preprocedural and postprocedural neurologic assessments (changes require immediate notification of neurosurgical team with the addition of head CT scan and possibly surgical intervention if necessary)[7]
- Invasive hemodynamic monitoring, with the addition of ICP monitoring via EVD

Acute Ischemic Stroke

If there is an AIS, patients within time guidelines, generally less than 3 hours of onset of symptoms, are given tissue plasminogen activator (tPA) to dissolve the thromboembolism.[1] If patients outside this therapeutic window present with symptoms of AIS, they are candidates for endovascular intervention. Of clinical importance, respiratory status must be evaluated, as a decrease in LOC may require endotracheal intubation and mechanical ventilation to protect the airway. Second to airway protection is hemodynamic stability. Maintenance of blood pressure is a goal for both anesthesia personnel in the intraoperative period and critical care nurses in the postoperative period. Hemodynamic stability is paramount to the preservation of neurologic function and must be closely monitored. It is strongly suggested to use intra-arterial blood pressure measurement for instant recognition of hemodynamic instability.[17] Hypertension is very common in patients presenting with AIS. Antihypertensive therapy to lower systolic blood pressure in a controlled manner to facilitate cerebral autoregulation and the maintenance of CPP must be considered.[1]

Nursing considerations
- Conduct hemodynamic monitoring to maintain blood pressure parameters postoperatively, with the common goals of systolic blood pressure greater than 140 mm Hg and less than 180 mm Hg.[1]
- Oversedation leading to airway obstruction and apnea can cause hypercarbia, leading to increased ICP and potential neurologic compromise.
- When tPA therapy is administered, monitor closely for bleeding; do not use anticoagulants within 24 hours of administration.[4]
- Closely monitor the surgical site (most commonly femoral) for hematoma formation and hemorrhage.
- The presence of hyperglycemia is associated with poor outcomes in neurosurgical patients and should be avoided.[1] The goal of serum glucose should be 70 to 140 mg/dL and greater than 50 mg/dL.[17]
- Maintain normothermia and particularly avoid hyperthermia with AIS.[10]

Subarachnoid Hemorrhage and Intracranial Aneurysms

Confirmation of the presence of aneurysms involves a complex workup, including diagnostic imaging studies. Commonly, aneurysms are the causative factor in spontaneous SAH.[1] Surgical clipping (via craniotomy) of intact aneurysms is still a widely practiced course of intervention. However, because of decreased morbidity and mortality, endovascular intervention, such as cerebral coiling and embolization, is preferred when appropriate.[1,5,7] During IR approaches in coiling cerebral aneurysm, anesthesia and nursing staff should always be prepared for the potentially fatal complication of severe hemorrhage. The standard of care should also include an available operating room on standby should emergent craniotomy be necessary for surgical clipping of the aneurysm to control hemorrhage.[13]

Nursing considerations for SAH
- Preoperative renal prophylaxis caused by the use of intravenous contrast and the risks associated for nephropathy[5]
- Placement of intra-arterial blood pressure monitoring and central line access for hemodynamic monitoring, fluid volume evaluation, and administration
- Postoperative monitoring of neuroendovascular access site at the groin

Cerebral Vasospasm

This highly mortal side effect of cerebral aneurysms/SAH requires the utmost vigilance from critical care nurses. Cerebral vasospasm (CVS) is a common side effect that typically presents within days 3 to 15 and up to day 21 after intervention.[1,7] CVS occurs because of many potential mechanisms of action that result in a narrowing of cerebral arteries leading to cerebral ischemia.[5] Current studies show that particularly delayed cerebral ischemia (DCI) can present with high morbidity, either with or without the presence of CVS.[18,19] In the neurointensive care unit, neurologic examinations must be conducted routinely to detect a deteriorating LOC that may indicate impending or ongoing CVS. DCI and CVS can be insidious in that they can present without an associated neurologic deficit. The routine use of transcranial Doppler (TCD) ultrasonography to denote areas of decreased blood flow is widely used.[7,19] The ability to detect DCI early and before CVS may lead to a decreased morbidity within this patient population.[19] The use of TCD ultrasonography in diagnosing CVS and DCI may also be advantageous in sedated patients when neurologic examinations are difficult to assess LOC.[7]

There are many aspects and methods of the treatment of CVS. Primarily, the implementation of triple H therapy (hypertension, hypervolemia, hemodilution [HHH]) and the oral administration of the calcium channel blocker nimodipine are considered the most effective.[20,21] Early interventions are associated with the best patient outcomes and improved prognosis.[20,22]

Patients that do not improve with HHH therapy should be considered for endovascular intervention.[5,18] Endovascular treatment of vasospasm via direct intra-arterial injection of vasodilators is quickly becoming a first-line treatment. Commonly vasodilators, such as nicardipine (calcium channel blocker) or papaverine, are used for intractable CVS unresponsive to HHH measures.[5,7] Typically patients are received from and returned to the ICU at the procedure conclusion. Critical care nursing is involved with the care throughout the course of therapeutic intervention. As with the SAH endovascular interventions, a thorough report from the anesthesia personnel directly involved in the patients' care must be obtained on transition of care after the procedure. GETA is the most common anesthesia for these cases. As anesthesia dissipates, the need for vasoactive and sedative medications may be required to prevent unwanted hypertension (HTN) and increased ICP. These effects are highly undesirable in recently treated patients with CVS.

Nursing considerations

- The goal of euvolemia is to prevent complications associated with hypervolemia.
- Administer both crystalloid and colloid to the goal central venous pressure (CVP).[5,7]
- Cardiopulmonary failure has been associated with aggressive fluid administration; thus, the implementation of hypervolemia has fallen out of favor.[1,7,22]
- Hypertension and the use of vasoactive infusions to increase blood pressure and, therefore, CPP are considered the most effective in HHH therapy.
- The hemodilution goal hematocrit levels are 30% to 35%.[20]

SUMMARY

The link between anesthesia and critical care nursing has profound implications in acute neurosurgical patients. Regardless of neurologic procedure or pathology, acute neurosurgical patients demand a heightened level of care. Critical care nurses are a fundamental presence to vigilantly assess for the most minute of changes in a patient's neurologic assessment and vital signs in the postsurgical arena. These neurologic changes may require an immediate response via nursing interventions and require an immediate notification of the surgical team to the presence of potential complications. Amid challenging disease processes and unique patient needs, the critical care nurse is undeniably the neurologic patients' advocate to ensure patient safety and promote a transition toward recovery.

REFERENCES

1. Hines R, Marschall K, editors. Stoelting's anesthesia and co-existing disease. 5th edition. Philadelphia: Churchill Livingstone/Elselvier; 2008.

2. Forsyth RJ, Wolny S, Rodrigues B. Routine intracranial pressure monitoring in acute coma. Cochrane Database Syst Rev 2010;(2):CD002043. http://dx.doi.org/10.1002/14651858.CD002043.pub2.
3. Bruder N, Ravussin P. Recovery from anesthesia and postoperative extubation of neurosurgical patients: a review. J Neurosurg Anesthesiol 1999;11(4):282–93.
4. Urden LD, Stacy KM, Lough ME. Thelan's critical care nursing diagnosis and management. 5th edition. St Louis (MO): Mosby; 2006.
5. Lin BF, Kuo CY, Wu ZF. Review of aneurysmal subarachnoid hemorrhage-Focus on treatment, anesthesia, cerebral vasospasm prophylaxis, and therapy. Acta Anaesthesiol Taiwan 2014;52:77–84.
6. Hart MG, Metcalfe SE, Grant R. Biopsy versus resection for high grade glioma. Cochrane Database Syst Rev 2014;(2):CD002034. http://dx.doi.org/10.1002/14651858.CD002034.
7. Bell R, Vo A, Veznedaroglu E, et al. The endovascular operating room as an extension of the intensive care unit: changing strategies in the management of neurovascular disease. Neurosurgery 2006;59(3):S56–65. http://dx.doi.org/10.1227/01.NEU.0000244733.85557.0E. Available at: www.neurosurgery-online.com. Accessed July 1, 2014.
8. Bruder N, Stordeur J, Ravussin P, et al. Metabolic and hemodynamic changes during recovery and tracheal extubation in neurosurgical patients: immediate versus delayed recovery. Anesth Analg 1999;89:674–8.
9. Milani WR, Antibas PL, Prado GF. Cooling for cerebral protection during brain surgery. Cochrane Database Syst Rev 2011;(10):CD006638. http://dx.doi.org/10.1002/14651858.CD006638.pub2.
10. Todd M, Hindman B, Clarke W, et al. Perioperative fever and outcome in surgical patients with aneurysmal subarachnoid hemorrhage. Neurosurgery 2009;64:897–908.
11. Dunbar P, Visco E, Lam A. Craniotomy procedures are associated with less analgesic requirements than other surgical procedures. Anesth Analg 1999;88:335–40.
12. Barr J, Fraser G, Puntillo K, et al. Clinical practice guidelines for the management of pain, agitation, and delirium in adult patients in the intensive care unit. Crit Care Med 2013;41:263–306.
13. Newfield P, Cottrell J, editors. Handbook of neuroanesthesia. 5th edition. Philadelphia: Lippincott Williams & Wilkins; 2012.
14. Tan C, Ries C, Mayson K, et al. Indication for surgery and the risk of postoperative nausea and vomiting after craniotomy: a case-control study. J Neurosurg Anesthesiol 2012;24:325–30.
15. Rowe S, Goodwin H, Brophy G, et al. Seizure prophylaxis in neurocritical care: a review of evidence-based support. Pharmacotherapy 2014;34(4):396–409. http://dx.doi.org/10.1002/phar.1374.
16. Hughey A, Lesniak M, Ansari S, et al. What will anesthesiologists be anesthetizing? Trends in neurosurgical procedure usage. Anesth Analg 2010;110:1686–97.
17. Talke P, Sharma D, Heyer E, et al. Society for Neuroscience in Anesthesiology and Critical Care expert consensus statement: anesthetic management of endovascular treatment for acute ischemic stroke. J Neurosurg Anesthesiol 2014;26:95–108.
18. Armonda R, Bell R, Vo A, et al. Wartime traumatic cerebral vasospasm: recent review of combat casualties. Neurosurgery 2006;59:1215–25.
19. Sarrafzadeh A, Vajkoczy P, Bijlenga P, et al. Monitoring in neurointensive care-the challenge to detect delayed cerebral ischemia in high-grade aneurysmal SAH. Front Neurol 2014;5:134. Available at: http://dx.doi.org/10.3389/fneur.2014.00134. Accessed July 1, 2014.

20. Adamczyk P, He S, Amar A, et al. Medical management of cerebral vasospasm following aneurysmal subarachnoid hemorrhage: a review of current and emerging therapeutic interventions. Neurol Res Int 2013;2013:462491. Available at: http://dx.doi.org/10.1155/2013/462491. Accessed July 1, 2014.
21. Valet G, Kimball M, Mocco J, et al. Vasospasm after aneurysmal subarachnoid hemorrhage: review of randomized controlled trials and meta-analysis in the literature. World Neurosurg 2011;76(5):446–54.
22. Kassell N, Peerless S, Durward Q, et al. Treatment of ischemic deficits from vasospasm with intravascular volume expansion and induced arterial hypertension. Neurosurgery 1982;11(3):337–43.

Massive Transfusion for Hemorrhagic Shock
What Every Critical Care Nurse Needs to Know

Susan Thibeault, MS, MBA, BSN, CRNA, EMT-P

KEYWORDS

- Massive transfusion • Red blood cell transfusion • Coagulopathy
- Hemorrhagic shock

KEY POINTS

- Protocol-driven therapy in massive transfusion benefits patients by:
  - ○ Individualized approach to resuscitation.
  - ○ Avoidance of iatrogenic coagulopathy by limiting crystalloid volumes.
  - ○ Early administration of packed red blood cells (PRBCs).
  - ○ Administering PRBCs with fresh frozen plasma and platelets in a 1:1:1 ratio.

HISTORY

Transfusions in the past were completed using whole blood until the development of blood component therapy in the 1980s. The advantages to blood component therapy are the storage time for each component individually is longer and resources are saved by administering only the portion of the blood that was required.[1]

Since the creation of blood component therapy, a patient with hypovolemia would receive packed red blood cells (PRBCs) and crystalloids, resulting in coagulopathies, and require additional blood components such as platelets (PLT) and fresh frozen plasma (FFP).

INTRODUCTION

Up until recently, the resuscitation for patients with hypovolemia, whether due to surgical losses or trauma, has been the early and aggressive administration of large amounts of crystalloid solutions. The use of high-volume crystalloid support is associated with increased hemorrhage and lower survival rates.[2–4] Recent studies indicate a survival benefit to protocol-driven transfusion strategies with specific ratios of

Disclosure Statement: The author has no conflicts of interest to declare.
Department of Anesthesiology, Yale-New Haven Hospital, 20 York Street, New Haven, CT 06510, USA
E-mail address: SusanThibeault@hotmail.com

Crit Care Nurs Clin N Am 27 (2015) 47–53
http://dx.doi.org/10.1016/j.cnc.2014.10.008
0899-5885/15/$ – see front matter © 2015 Elsevier Inc. All rights reserved.

PRBCs, FFP, and PLT. Protocol-driven therapy in massive transfusion also reduces intensive care unit and hospital lengths of stay, decreased ventilator-dependent days, and overall patient care costs.[5,6]

Massive transfusion is defined as complete replacement of a patient's blood volume or approximately 10 units of PRBCs within a 24-hour period or one red blood cells (RBC) volume in 24 hours for a pediatric patient.[7] This article reviews the most recent understanding and recommendations in massive transfusion along with the unintended consequences in the management of patients with profound hemorrhage.

Although the focus of this journal series is "critical care nursing in the operating room," research on massive transfusion and the resulting protocols has been derived from research studies not only in the surgical setting but also in the field of trauma medicine, most specifically in the military battlefields. The research referenced in this article is not exclusive to the operating room environment, but rather the entire realm of critical care.

TREATMENT

The primary goal of resuscitation is restoration of cellular perfusion. A 2-pronged approach should be used when caring for a patient in hemorrhagic hypovolemic shock. Initially, aggressive efforts should be made to stop blood loss, which in the surgical and trauma settings can pose a challenge. Second, replacing fluid volume deficits, oxygen-carrying capacity, and coagulation factors should be addressed.

IDEAL RATIO/FLUID RESUSCITATION

The approach to volume resuscitation is individualized based on the clinical condition of the patient, anticipated further hemorrhagic losses (or achievement of hemostasis), and comorbidities. Crystalloid intravenous (IV) fluids are used initially in resuscitation. IV fluid administration should be guided by evidence of adequate end-organ perfusion such as adequate urine output for weight and lactate less than 2.0. It is a fine balance maintaining the need for tissue perfusion and the risk of worsening bleeding through excess pressure on hemostatic clots and the induction of coagulopathy.

In general, for adult trauma patients with bleeding and without brain injury, a systolic blood pressure between 80 and 100 mm Hg is considered reasonable until bleeding has been controlled.[8,9] In trauma patients with a concomitant traumatic brain injury, a cerebral perfusion pressure of at least 60 mm Hg should be maintained to avoid cerebral hypoperfusion. Cerebral hypoperfusion in the setting of brain trauma is associated with a significant worsening in outcomes and must be avoided.[10]

TRANSFUSION AND MASSIVE TRANSFUSION
Packed Red Blood Cells

In contrast to crystalloid IV resuscitation, fluid replacement with PRBCs provides volume, osmotic pressure, and oxygen-carrying capacity. Transfusion is indicated to maintain a hemoglobin level between 7 and 9 g/dL. Type-specific blood should be administered if available. However, if type-specific blood is not available, type O RhD-negative PRBCs are recommended, especially for the parturient, to prevent development of anti-D antibodies.

PRBCs are prepared by removing most of the plasma from citrated whole blood. Actual changes depend on the state of hydration and the rate of bleeding. Because most of the plasma has been removed, PRBCs cause fewer transfusion and allergic reactions than whole blood does.[11] A general rule of thumb is that a single unit of

PRBCs increases the hemoglobin by 1 g/dL and hematocrit by 2% to 3%. In pediatric patients, there is an approximate increase in hematocrit of 1% for each 1 mL/kg of packed cells. For example, if 5 mL/kg of PRBCs is transfused, the hematocrit will increase by approximately 5%.[12]

Banked PRBCs changes that occur are important for the critical care nurse to be aware of and include the following:

- Depletion of 2,3-diphosphoglycerate (this controls how easily a RBC lets go of the oxygen it is carrying at the tissue level; decreased amounts of this led to decreased oxygen delivery at the tissue level)
- Depletion of adenosine triphosphate (the energy for metabolism)
- Oxidative damage
- Increased adhesion to vascular epithelium
- Altered RBC morphology (changes in shape, membrane loss, and decreased flexibility)
- Microaggregate accumulation
- Hyperkalemia (may be as elevated as 17.2 mEg/L)
- Hemolysis
- Absence of factors V and VII
- Accumulation of proinflammatory metabolic and breakdown products[12]

In addition, banked PRBCs contain the preservative sodium citrate, which binds calcium, causing hypocalcemia, which has a 2-fold effect: it inhibits coagulation (because calcium is a key component to the extrinsic clotting cascade) and contributes to hypoperfused state (as calcium plays a key role in smooth muscle contraction in the blood vessels).[13]

As the amounts of PRBC transfusion increase, the risks for coagulopathy increase. Research has demonstrated that there are benefits from the empiric administration of FFP and PLT in addition to the PRBCs.[14] Whole-blood resuscitation is common and effective in the setting of military operations but is impractical in the civilian hospital environment.

Fresh Frozen Plasma

FFP contains all coagulation factors and can be used to reverse the anticoagulant effects of medications that affect the extrinsic clotting pathway (ie, warfarin), correction of coagulopathy, and correction of dilutional coagulopathy.[13]

Platelets

Platelets are essential in achieving hemostasis by forming the "platelet plug" and, without PLT, hemostasis is not possible. Platelet transfusion is indicated in the setting of acute blood loss, dilutional coagulopathy, and platelet dysfunction, for example, in the setting of chronic aspirin or clopidodrel therapy.[13]

A unit of whole blood has a volume of about 500 mL, a hematocrit of about 40%, PLT of about 175,000, and approximately 1500 mg of fibrinogen. Transfusion in a 1:1:1 strategy provides 660 mL of volume, a hematocrit of 29%, 87,000 PLT, and 750 mg of fibrinogen, as compared with the absence of PLT and fibrinogen in simple PRBC transfusion. Conceptually, this approach will proactively decrease the incidence of coagulopathy associated with shock states and transfusion. The ideal ratio, however, has not been determined and is still the source of debate among experts in trauma care and resuscitation. Most massive transfusion protocols have a PRBC:FFP:PLT ratio somewhere between 2:1:1 and 1:1:1.[8,15,16] **Table 1** summarizes

Table 1 Whole blood transfusion compared with massive transfusion		
	Whole Blood	1:1:1 Massive Transfusion
Volume (mL)	500	660
Hematocrit (%)	40	29
Platelet count	175,000	87,000
Fibrinogen (mg)	1500	750

the differences between whole blood transfusion and massive transfusion using a 1:1:1 strategy.

Additional Volume Expanders and Medications

There has been little success in the development of artificial hemoglobin products and non-oxygen-carrying colloids.

Tranexamic acid may be useful in managing coagulopathy used in conjunction with massive transfusion protocols. Tranexamic acid is a synthetic agent that inhibits plasmin and plasminogen by preserving clots as an antifibrinolytic. A worldwide civilian trauma study and military trauma data suggest that the administration of tranexamic acid improves outcomes in trauma patients who require massive transfusion. As with blood product ratios, however, there is still disagreement about the role of tranexamic acid as well as concerns regarding the associated prothrombic risk of administration. Aminocaproic acid is a similar agent that may be used; however, it possesses about one-tenth the antifibrinolytic effect.[17–19]

RISKS/ADVERSE OUTCOMES
Transfusion Coagulopathy

Resuscitation paradoxically contributes to coagulopathy through clotting factor consumption, clotting factor dilution, and the replacement of volume with PRBCs and IV fluids that have no clotting factors. Dilutional thrombocytopenia is a complication of massive transfusion because of dilution of the patient's own PLT. In addition, there may be coagulation pathway derangements associated with acidosis and hypothermia. Laboratory studies are of limited value in the actively hemorrhaging patient. Standard prothrombin time, partial thromboplastin time, and international normalized ratio (INR) testing evaluate only the first 4% of thrombin production and must be supplemented by evaluation of fibrinogen and platelet values. When the INR exceeds 1.5, FFP transfusion of at least 15 mL/kg is indicated. The administration of an apheresis pack of PLT should be considered when the platelet count is less than 50 to 100 $\times$ 10^9/L, and cryoprecipitate to replete clotting factors VIII, XIII, von Willebrand factor, and fibrinogen should be considered when the measured fibrinogen is less than 1.5 to 2 g/dL. Thromboelastography offers greater information to guide coagulopathy management than do laboratory values but is not currently in widespread clinical use.[8,15,16]

Disseminated Intravascular Coagulation

Disseminated intravascular coagulation (DIC) may play a secondary role in posttransfusion hemorrhage. Factors V and VIII are limited in stored blood and absent in units of PRBCs. Fibrinogen is absent in packed cells. A deficiency of most clotting factors, especially factors V and VIII and fibrinogen, occurs with massive transfusions. This deficiency is a form of consumptive coagulopathy, meaning the intrinsic clotting factors have been used in an attempt to halt hemorrhage, leaving a deficiency of clotting factors, which contributes to continued blood losses.[11]

Risks/Complications

All transfusions are associated with risks, and the risks are exacerbated by massive transfusion. Clinicians should be attentive for the development of hypocalcemia, hyperkalemia, acidosis, hypothermia, and the risk of pulmonary dysfunction known as transfusion-related acute lung injury (TRALI).[17,18]

TRALI refers to noncardiogenic pulmonary edema occurring during or shortly after the transfusion of blood products. A leading cause of transfusion-related mortality and morbidity, TRALI has been reported to occur in as many as 3% of patients receiving transfusions.[11]

RBC transfusion is associated with risks for infection, lung injury, acidosis, electrolyte derangement, and hypothermia. The administration of older units of banked blood may do little to improve oxygen delivery. Once bleeding is controlled, it is clear that a restrictive transfusion strategy of tolerating a hemoglobin of 7 g/dL is associated with markedly improved outcomes and mortality.[8,15,20,21]

Manage Existing Coagulopathy

Patients may be on a regimen of acute or chronic anticoagulant medications. In the setting of uncontrolled hemorrhage, treating an existing coagulopathy will contribute to early hemostasis and a decreased need for resuscitation. Management varies with the agent used.[8,15,16]

Warfarin can be reversed with the administration of FFP and the administration of vitamin K. Uncrossmatched FFP is type AB and should be given in a dose of at least 15 mL/kg of actual body weight. IV vitamin K administration is recommended for warfarin reversal in patients with acute bleeding. It should be given by slow IV infusion, and clinicians should remember that there is a remote risk of anaphylactoid reaction to vitamin K. For patients with life-threatening bleeding from warfarin, the prothrombin complex concentrates (PCC) are also an option for rapid reversal. These agents contain varying amounts of factors II, IX, and X. Some contain factor VII and proteins C and S. They reverse an elevated INR much more rapidly than do FFP and vitamin K and are associated with decreased intracranial hematoma volume expansion in patients with elevated INR and intercranial hemorrhage. There has yet to be a demonstration of improved patient outcome with PCC use, however.

Protamine is effective, to varying degrees, as a reversal agent for heparin, low-molecular-weight heparins, and factor Xa inhibitors. There is approximately a risk that 0.2% of patients who receive protamine will have an anaphylactic reaction.

The direct thrombin inhibitors are not amenable to reversal with FFP, vitamin K, factor VII concentrate, or the PCC agents.

Last, many patients are on a regimen of aspirin. Aspirin irreversibly blocks cyclooxygenase, the enzyme that catalyzes the conversion of arachidonic acid to thromboxane A2. This inhibition of platelet aggregation lasts for the entire 10-day lifespan of the platelet. There is a lack of consensus on how to manage preinjury aspirin use in patients with significant traumatic or surgical bleeding. There is a lack of evidence that platelet administration is warranted under these circumstances.

SUMMARY

Recent research has demonstrated that early implementation of protocol-driven massive resuscitation strategies improves patient survival and decreases the lengths of stay and the number of ventilator-dependent days. The implementation of massive transfusion protocols has a significant impact on patient outcomes. Nurses play an important role in recognizing the need for implementation of massive transfusion protocols, to anticipate and manage the potential risks and adverse outcomes, and to assess for the key indicators of adequate resuscitation efforts.

REFERENCES

1. Zink KA, Sambasivan CN, Holcomb JB, et al. A high ratio of platelets to packed red blood cells in the first 6 hours of massive transfusion improves outcomes in a large multicenter study. Am J Surg 2009;197:565–70.
2. Kowalenko T, Stern S, Dronen S, et al. Improved outcome with hypotensive resuscitation of uncontrolled hemorrhagic shock in a swine model. J Trauma 1992;33: 349–53.
3. Balogh Z, McKinley BA, Holcomb JB, et al. Both primary and secondary abdominal compartment syndrome can be predicted early and are harbingers of multiple organ failure. J Trauma 2003;54:848–59.
4. Joshi GP. Intraoperative fluid restriction improves outcome after major elective gastrointestinal surgery. Anesth Analg 2005;101:601–5.
5. Riskin DJ, Tsai TC, Riskin L, et al. Massive transfusion protocols: the role of aggressive resuscitation versus product ratio in mortality reduction. J Am Coll Surg 2009;209:198–205.
6. Young PP, Cotton BA, Goodnough LT. Massive transfusion protocols for patients with substantial hemorrhage. Transfus Med Rev 2011;25:293–303.
7. Malone DL, Hess JR, Fingerhut A. Massive transfusion practices around the globe and a suggestion for a common massive transfusion protocol. J Trauma 2006;60:S91–6.
8. Bhananker S, Ramaiah R. Trends in trauma resuscitation. Int J Crit Illn Inj Sci 2011;1:51–6.
9. Trauma, American College of Surgeons (A. C. o. S. C. o.). Advanced trauma life support for doctors student course manual. 9th edition. Glen Rock, PA: Hearthside Publishing Services; 2012.
10. Medicine, Society of Critical Care Medicine (S. o. C. C.). Fundamental critical care support. 5th edition. 2012.
11. Gorgas DL, Kaide CG. Hapter 28: Transfusion therapy: blood and blood products. In: Roberts JR, Custalow CB. Clinical procedures in emergency medicine. Philadelphia: Elsevier Saunders; 6th edition. 2014. p. 496–578.
12. Morgan GE, Mitchell MS, Murphy MJ, et al. Fluid management and transfusion. Clinical Anesthesiology. New York: Lange Medical Books/McGraw-Hill Medical Publishing Division; 4th edition. 2006. p. 690–707.
13. Lynn RR, Winner LA. Ch 20: Fluids, electrolytes, and blood component therapy. Nurse Anesth 2013;382–402.
14. Inaba K, Lustenberger T, Rhee P, et al. The impact of platelet transfusion in massively transfused trauma patients. J Am Coll Surg 2010;211:573–9.
15. Napolitano L, Kurek S, Luchette F, et al. Clinical practice guideline: red blood cell transfusion in adult trauma and critical care. J Trauma 2009;67(6): 1439–42.
16. Roissaint R, Bouillon B, Cerny V, et al. Management of bleeding following major trauma: an updated European guideline. Crit Care 2010;14:852–82.
17. Morrison J, Dubrose J, Rasmussen T, et al. Military application of tranexamic acid in trauma emergency resuscitation study. Arch Surg 2012;147(2):113–9.

18. Shakur H, Roberts I, Bautista R, et al. Effect of tranexamic acid on death, vascular occlusive events, and blood transfusion with significant hemorrhage: a randomised, placebo-controlled trial. Lancet 2010;376(9734):23–32.
19. Valle E, Allen C, Van Haren R, et al. Do all trauma patients benefit from tranexamic acid? J Trauma Acute Care Surg 2014;76(6):1373–8.
20. Gajic O. Transfusion related acute lung injury in the critically ill. Am J Respir Crit Care Med 2007;176:866–90.
21. Netzer G. Association of RBC transfusion with mortality in patients with acute lung injury. Chest 2007;132:1116–21.

Management of the Difficult Airway

Larissa Galante, CRNA, MSN

KEYWORDS

- Airway management • Difficult airway • Intubation • Extubation • Airway algorithm

KEY POINTS

- Patients with a difficult airway present unique challenges and considerations.
- It is recommended that clinicians assess patients for a possible difficult airway by obtaining a thorough history and physical examination.
- Familiarity with difficult airway management guidelines, algorithms, tools, and techniques is essential to formulating a safe and effective plan for intubation as well as extubation of patients with this condition.

MANAGEMENT OF THE DIFFICULT AIRWAY

Airway management skills are critical to caring for patients in any setting. The American Society of Anesthesiologists defines a difficult airway as an airway in which an experienced anesthesia provider encounters difficulty with face mask ventilation, difficulty with tracheal intubation, or both.[1] The realm of airway management has advanced significantly in the last 15 years as various devices, tools, techniques, pharmaceuticals, and algorithms have been developed and implemented successfully. Although with careful planning an expertise in a limited number of tools is sufficient in most situations, the variety of options can be overwhelming.[2] Several detailed publications exist regarding techniques and specifications of airway equipment and tools. This article will focus on airway evaluation, identification, planning, extubation, and care of the patient with a difficult airway.

PREPARATION

Formulating a plan for management of the difficult airway is essential for success. The major adverse outcomes associated with a difficult airway include brain injury, cardiopulmonary arrest, need for surgical airway, trauma to the teeth and airway,

Disclosure: No compensation has been received from any company for the content in this article.
Department of Anesthesiology, Yale-New Haven Hospital, 20 York Street, New Haven, CT 06510, USA
E-mail address: Larissagalante@hotmail.com

and death. Many factors influence planning including the condition of the patient, the anticipated procedure, and the skills and preferences of the practitioner who will be managing the airway. Whether the difficult airway presents in the perioperative, intensive care, or emergency setting, following sentence.[1,2]

Several basic preparations should be taken for difficult airway management[1,2]:

1. Availability of a portable cart or storage unit with specialized equipment
2. Informing the patient or person responsible of the unique related risks and procedures
3. Availability of another individual capable of assisting during airway management
4. Preoxygenation of the patient, when possible, prior to initiating management of the airway; this may be limited in uncooperative or pediatric patients
5. Administration of supplemental oxygen throughout the airway management process, such as via nasal cannula, facemask, blow by, laryngeal mask airway (LMA), insufflation, and other available methods

The Difficult Airway Algorithm (DAA) (**Fig. 1**)[1] of the American Society of Anesthesiologists (ASA) is the foundation of the practice of difficult airway management. It provides clinicians with a decision path to choose when dealing with an anticipated difficult airway, a "can't intubate but can ventilate situation," and the "can't intubate/can't ventilate scenario."

The following are 4 choices for management:

1. Awake intubation versus anesthetized intubation
   ■ Lack of cooperation or a pediatric patient can be a limiting factor in the options for awake intubation; using an approach that would not be considered as a primary method in a cooperative patient may be necessary
2. Noninvasive techniques versus invasive techniques
3. Video-assisted laryngoscopy as the primary approach to intubation
4. Maintenance of spontaneous ventilation versus halting of spontaneous ventilation

A report by Rosenblatt[3] describes an airway approach algorithm (AAA) to organize airway related information prior to anesthetizing the patient, and this is intended to lead the clinician to choosing the best entryway to the DAA in order to avoid the emergency branch. If airway control fails, the emergency branch of the algorithm should be used by default. The AAA considers 6 basic problems identified by the ASA that may be encountered with a difficult airway including difficulty with patient cooperation or consent, mask ventilation, supraglottic airway placement, laryngoscopy, intubation, and surgical airway access.[1,3]

Is Airway Control Necessary?

Consider the surgical procedure, surgeon, skills of the anesthesia provider, and patient cooperation. Using regional anesthesia or local infiltration with or without sedation has potential to require manipulation of the airway or conversion to a general anesthetic. Although it may provide an alternative to direct management of difficult airway, it is not a definitive solution and does not eliminate the need for a strategic plan for intubating a difficult airway.[1–3]

Is There Potential for a Difficult Laryngoscopy?

Laryngoscopy is the standard of care and is also the quickest route to achieving tracheal intubation by most skilled practitioners. Review of the patient's history and a physical examination provide valuable information in assessing the potential for difficult laryngoscopy. Clinical experience plays a large role in this assessment. If the

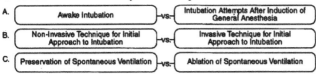

DIFFICULT AIRWAY ALGORITHM

1. Assess the likelihood and clinical impact of basic management problems:
   A. Difficult Ventilation
   B. Difficult Intubation
   C. Difficulty with Patient Cooperation or Consent
   D. Difficult Tracheostomy

2. Actively pursue opportunities to deliver supplemental oxygen throughout the process of difficult airway management

3. Consider the relative merits and feasibility of basic management choices:

   A. Awake Intubation –vs– Intubation Attempts After Induction of General Anesthesia

   B. Non-Invasive Technique for Initial Approach to Intubation –vs– Invasive Technique for Initial Approach to Intubation

   C. Preservation of Spontaneous Ventilation –vs– Ablation of Spontaneous Ventilation

4. Develop primary and alternative strategies:

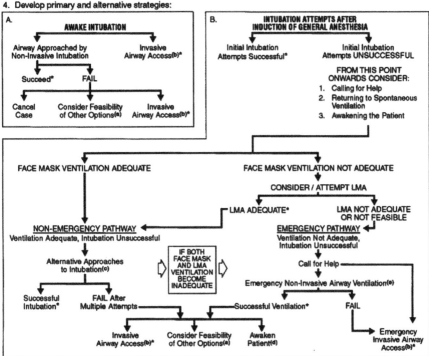

* Confirm ventilation, tracheal intubation, or LMA placement with exhaled CO_2

a. Other options include (but are not limited to): surgery utilizing face mask or LMA anesthesia, local anesthesia infiltration or regional nerve blockade. Pursuit of these options usually implies that mask ventilation will not be problematic. Therefore, these options may be of limited value if this step in the algorithm has been reached via the Emergency Pathway.

b. Invasive airway access includes surgical or percutaneous tracheostomy or cricothyrotomy.

c. Alternative non-invasive approaches to difficult intubation include (but are not limited to): use of different laryngoscope blades, LMA as an intubation conduit (with or without fiberoptic guidance), fiberoptic intubation, intubating stylet or tube changer, light wand, retrograde intubation, and blind oral or nasal intubation.

d. Consider re-preparation of the patient for awake intubation or canceling surgery.

e. Options for emergency non-invasive airway ventilation include (but are not limited to): rigid bronchoscope, esophageal-tracheal combitube ventilation, or transtracheal jet ventilation.

Fig. 1. Difficult airway algorithm. (*From* Apfelbaum JL, Hagberg CA, Caplan RA, et al. Practice guidelines for management of the difficult airway: an updated report by the American Society of Anesthesiologists Task Force on Management of the Difficult Airway. Anesthesiology 2013;118(2):251–70; with permission.)

answer to this question is "no," and intubation becomes difficult, the DAA should be followed.

Can Supralaryngeal Ventilation Be Used?

If ventilation can be achieved by supraglottic airways such as an LMA, a variety of laryngeal tubes, or mask, consequence of failed intubation is not emergent. With an uncooperatvive patient, spontaneous ventilation with inhaled anesthesia may be a viable option.

Is the Stomach Empty?

Patients not considered to have an empty stomach should not receive ventilation via supralaryngeal devices due to the risk of regurgitation as a result of increased gastric pressures from distension. Patients at risk for aspiration or full stomach who present with difficulty to intubate should be treated in the "cannot intubate and cannot venti-late" branch of the DAA, and awake management should be considered.

Will the Patient Tolerate a Period of Apnea?

Adult patients who are healthy and adequately preoxygenated should tolerate apneic periods of 5 to 9 minutes. Healthy and adequately preoxygenated children should be able to tolerate apneic periods of 2 to 4 minutes. Premature oxyhemoglobin desatura-tion may occur in the obese, parturient, or clinically ill patients as well as in patients who are inadequately preoxygenated. Apneic periods after induction may range from 30 to 60 seconds or 4 to 7 minutes if succinylcholine is given.

AIRWAY EVALUATION

Recognition of a potentially difficult airway requires a thorough and comprehensive evaluation. The goal is to assess for medical, surgical, and anesthetic elements that may indicate the presence of a difficult airway. A variety of conditions and diseases exist which have significant implication for the anatomy and physiology of the airway (**Table 1**).

In the history, a variety of questions should be asked:

- Does the patient have a known history of difficult airway?
- Has the patient awoken with an extremely sore throat, oropharyngeal bleeding, or difficulty breathing after previous surgery?
- Is the patient presenting with trauma, burns, or for current/past major neck or upper airway surgery?
- Is the patient obese, morbidly obese, or have obstructive sleep apnea?
- Does the patient have arthritis, especially rheumatoid arthritis, or autoimmune disease such as scleroderma?
- Does the patient have any airway or head/neck tumors, infections, or history of radiation?
- Is there a history of any syndromes, particularly congenital?
- Is the patient at risk for aspiration?

Obesity and Obstructive Sleep Apnea

The Centers for Disease Control and Prevention defines obesity as body mass index (BMI) greater than 30 kg/m^2.[4] Obstructive sleep apnea (OSA) is a syndrome in which periodic, partial, or complete obstruction of upper airway occurs during sleep, and as many as 71% of morbidly obese patient have this condition, which is marked by a

Table 1
Factors associated with difficult airway

Congenital Syndromes	
Alpert syndrome	Hypoplasia of maxilla, cleft soft palate, tracheobronchial anomalies of cartilage
Beckwith syndrome	Macroglossia
Cherubism	Maxillary and mandibular tumorous lesions with intraoral masses.
Cretinism	Absence of thyroid tissue or defect in thyroxine synthesis, macroglossia, goiter, tracheal compression, laryngeal, or tracheal deviation
Pierre-Robin syndrome	Micrognathia, macroglossia, cleft soft palate, glossoptosis
Treacher-Collins syndrome	Malar and mandibular hypoplasia, auricular and ocular defects, choanal atresia
Goldenhar syndrome	Malar and mandibular hypoplasia, auricular and ocular defects, occipitalization of atlas
Down syndrome	Macroglosia, bridge of the nose poorly developed, or absent, atlantooxipital instability and other cervical spine abnormalities, microcephaly
Kippel-Feil	Congenital fusion of variable number of cervical vertebrae, restricted movement
Goiter	Tracheal compression, deviation of larynx or trachea
Infections	
Supragolottitis, epiglottis, and croup	Can cause laryngeal edema
Abscesses, Ludwig's angina	In any part of the airway can cause distortion and trismus
Arthritis (rheumatoid, ankylosing spondylitis)	Temporomandibular joint stiffness, cricoarytenoid arthritis, laryngeal deviation, limited cervical spine mobility
Tumors, benign or malignant tumors	Can cause stenosis or distortion of the airway, fixation of larynx or adjacent tissues due to infiltration due to fibrosis or radiation, and also airway edema
Obesity	Short thick neck, oropharyngeal redundant tissue, sleep apnea
Trauma	Airway edema, hematoma, untable fractures of cervical spine, mandible, and vertebrae, pneumothorax
Acromegaly	Macroglossia, prognathism
Lingual-tonsil hypertrophy or hyperplasia	Can cause displacement of epiglottis and occupy vallecula[6]

Data from Refs.[2,5,6]

higher incidence of difficult mask ventilation, higher risk pulmonary aspiration, airway obstruction, and rapid oxygen desaturation after induction. Approximately 7.5% of morbidly obese patients have reported difficult intubation. An additional concern is the higher susceptibility to respiratory-depressant effects of opioids and anesthetics as well as an increased risk of hypoxia requiring continuous positive airway pressure (CPAP) treatment. Positioning these patients requires additional attention.

Rheumatoid Arthritis

Patients with this disease decreased neck mobility and anatomic abnormalities. Laryngeal involvement in rheumatoid arthritis is 13% to 75% in clinical studies and 45% to 88% in postmortem studies. Larynx deviation and arthritis of cricoarytenoid joints and laryngeal rheumatoid nodules are worsened by microtrauma, and fiberoptic intubation should be chosen.

Aspiration Risk

Patients who are at risk for pulmonary aspiration of gastric contents include those who;

Are nonfasting or coughing after eating or drinking,
Have delayed gastric emptying due to systemic disease such as diabetes, postvagotomy, collagen vascular disease, Parkinson disease, thyroid dysfunction, liver disease, central nervous system tumors, chronic renal insufficiency, voice changes, vocal cord polyps, or pneumonia, acute narcotic therapy, trauma, intensive care unit admission
Are pregnant (gestational age $\geq$12 weeks) and immediate postpartum patients
Have poorly controlled reflux.[3]

PHYSICAL EXAMINATION

The Mallampati evaluation correlates tongue size to pharyngeal size (**Fig. 2**). It is performed with the patient in sitting position, head neutral, mouth wide open, and tongue maximally protruded. Classification assignment depends on the extent to which the base of tongue affects visibility of pharyngeal structures.[7] In 1987, Samsoon and Youn modified this classification to include a fourth class. This test is an indirect means to evaluate the proportion of the tongue relative to the oropharynx.[5]

The Cormack and Lehane scale describes views of the vocal cords upon laryngoscopy (**Fig. 3**). Another acronym used for airway assessment that includes several of the examinations in **Table 2** is the LEMON[5] airway assessment; 1 point is given for each of the following criteria for a maximum of 10 points. Difficult intubation patients have higher scores (**Fig. 4**).

L = Look externally for facial trauma, large incisors, facial hair, large tongue
E = Evaluate the 3-2-2 rule

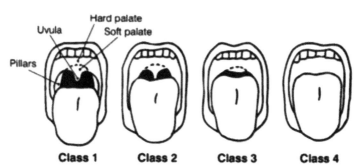

Fig. 2. The mallampati test. Class 1. Complete visualization of the soft palate. Class 2. Complete visualization of the uvula. Class 3. Visualization of only the base of the uvula. Class 4. Soft palate is not visible at all. (*From* Mallampati S. Clinical assessment of airway. Anesthesiol Clin North America 1995;13(2):301–6; with permission.)

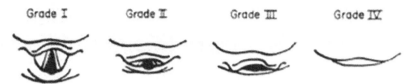

Fig. 3. Cormack and Lehane grade views in laryngoscopy. Grade 1. visualization of entire laryngeal aperture. Grade 2. Visualization of only posterior commissure of laryngeal aperture. Grade 3. Visualization of only epiglottis. Grade 4. Visualization of just the soft palate. (*From* Samsoon GL, Young JR. Difficult tracheal intubation: a retrospective study. Anaesthesia 1987;42(5):487–90; with permission.)

3 finger breadth incisor distance
3 finger breadth hyoid–mental distance
2 finger breadth thyroid to mouth distance
M = Mallampatti greater than 3
O = Obstruction such as abscess, epiglottitis, trauma
N = Neck mobility limitation

METHODS AND TOOLS FOR INTUBATION

Awake intubation is recommended for patients with identified difficult airways. Use of a fiberoptic bronchoscope is successful in 88% to 100% of these patients, although other tools such as intubation through supraglottic devices, glidescope, and other tools have been used successfully. Patient cooperation may be limiting factor.[1]

The fiberoptic bronchoscope is a difficult technique to learn and master, and unless used frequently, competency may be difficult to maintain. Proficiency in difficult airway management is determined by mastering several techniques, which may be useful in solving potential difficulties in various situations. A contraindication to using the fiberoptic bronchoscope is inexperience in using the technique.[8] Additional oxygen can be delivered through the suction channel, and this scope can be used in conjunction with other devices such as the glidescope.

Video-assisted laryngoscopy provides improved laryngeal views, higher success with first attempt, and greater frequency of successful intubation than with direct laryngoscopy.[1] The McGrath Series 5 video laryngoscopy has been used successfully in awake intubations in a randomized clinical trial.[9] It can improve visualization of glottis structures 1 or 2 grades in the Cormack Lehane classification system (**Fig. 3**) compared with the Macintosh blade. The Mcgrath video laryngoscope has been used as a rescue technique in cases of unexpected management of a difficult airway, and a case series has been published.[8]

Intubating stylets or tube changers are also an option and can be used successfully for difficult intubations. Mild mucosal bleeding and sore throat are complications associated with stylets, and lung laceration and gastric perforation are associated with exchange catheters.[1] A lighted stylet such as the light wand utilizes transillumination of tissue in the anterior neck to guide the tip of the endotracheal tube. This is a blind technique and should not be applied in order to avoid trauma.[10]

Supraglottic airways such as the LMA have shown to be rescue devices in patients who cannot be intubated or mask ventilated. The LMA can be used with a fiberoptic bronchoscope for intubation, and can maintain or restore ventilation in the difficult airway patient.[11] Supraglottic devices do have a risk of bronchospasm, respiratory

Table 2
Physical examination

Physical Examination	Nonreassuring Finding
Patency of nares	Masses in nasal cavity, deviated septum, and polyps
Interincisor gap or distance	<2 large finger breadths or 3 cm between upper and lower incisors
Teeth	Prominent, long incisors or overbite can limit the alignment of oral and pharyngeal axes during laryngoscopy Edentulous patient may experience hypopharyngeal tongue obstruction
Upper lip bite test relationship of maxillary and mandibular incisors	Inability to protrude mandibular incisors in front of maxillary incisors
Palate shape	High arch or long narrow mouth
Temporomandubular mobility and mouth opening	Small mouth opening, lockjaw, TMJ pain
Submental space—hyomental and thyromental	Should be >6 cm
Neck	Short thick neck, masses, limited atlantooccipital joint extension, inability to touch tip of chin to chest
Voice	Abnormalities, hoarseness, stridor, tracheostomy scar, possible stenosis
Body habitus	Body mass index above 25
Physiologic conditions	Pregnancy and obesity
Mandibular space	Stiff, occupied by mass, indurated
Thyromental distance- distance from the thyroid notch to the mentum with full extension of patient's neck.	<6 cm or 3 finger breadth in adults >6.5 cm is normal Alignment of laryngeal-pharyngeal axis may be difficult if this distance is short
Sternomental distancefrom supersternal notch to mentum	Value of <12 cm predicts difficult intubation.
Mandibulo–hyoid distance—length from chin to hyoid.	<4 cm or 3 finger breadths; as vertical distance from mandible to hyoid increases, laryngoscopy becomes more difficult
Visibility of uvula	Not visible when patient protrudes tongue in sitting position (see **Fig. 2**)
Systemic disease	Respiratory failure, coronary artery disease, acromegaly, arthritis, obesity, obstructive sleep apnea
Beard and facial hair	Beard may impede creating proper seal or disguise underlying abnormality like a disfiguring malignancy
Body jewelry	Piercing of lips, tongue, check, chin, eyebrows, ear can present risk for aspiration, tearing, bleeding, or trauma to the airway

Abbreviation: TMJ, temporomandibular joint.

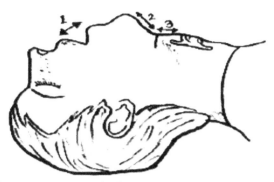

Fig. 4. LEMON airway assessment method; 1 = Inter-incisor distance in fingers, 2 = Hyoid mental distance in fingers, 3 = Thyroid to floor of mouth in fingers.

obstruction, laryngeal nerve injury, edema, and hypoglossal nerve paralysis when used in difficult patient. Laryngeal/pharyngeal tumor patients have been successfully ventilated with laryngeal tubes.[1]

Cricothyrotomy is the end point of the difficult airway algorithm. It is a lifesaving procedure that involves accessing the airway via the cricothyroid membrane.[11] This technique is applicable to patients in all settings from before hospital entry, emergency room, perioperative, and intensive care. The percutaneous technique uses the Seldinger technique to guide the endotracheal tube or tracheostomy device into the trachea.

A tracheostomy is a secure airway established below the level of the cricoid cartilage. This technique may be used emergently in children younger than 10 years or in individuals with altered or distorted airway anatomy, such as due to tumors or infection, if airway loss occurs. It is often the preferred technique in patients undergoing extensive neck surgery. The patient is intubated, and then a surgical tracheostomy is placed.[11]

Extubation

Extubation of the difficult airway patient is an important part of airway management. Just as with intubation, a plan is essential to patient safety, as significant morbidity and mortality are associated with extubation. Following the implementation of the difficult airway management guidelines by the ASA, closed claims database analysis showed a decrease in claims of death and brain death with induction and intubation, but there was no decrease of these occurrences with emergence, extubation, and postoperative course.[2,12] According to the NAP4 study and the ASA closed claims databases, poor outcomes were attributed to "less than appropriate care or judgment," presence of head and neck pathologies or postsurgical changes, and incomplete handoff communications and lack of adequate postoperative monitoring. Approximately 30% of events occurred because of poor airway management strategies, inadequate assessment of risk factors for difficult airway, and overall failure to plan.

As with intubation, developing a plan depends upon the surgery, state of the patient, and the preferences and skills of the anesthesia provider.[1] In order to plan for successful extubation, several steps should be taken[1,2,12]:

1. Preemptive optimization of patient conditions
2. Careful timing of extubation
3. Presence of experienced personnel trained in advanced airway management

4. Availability of necessary equipment and appropriate postextubation monitoring
5. Identification of patient who may have difficult airway
6. Recognition of situations at increased risk postextubation airway compromise
7. Understanding of causes and underlying mechanisms of extubation failure

At-risk extubation is a category describing a situation in which there may be questionable ability to maintain the airway after removal of the endotracheal tube. Scenarios that fall into this description are patients with difficult intubations, full stomachs, hemodynamic instability, acid–base imbalance, and poor temperature control.[12] General clinical factors that may produce adverse impact on ventilation should be identified, as well as a plan in the event that the patient cannot maintain adequate ventilation after extubation.[13] A strategy for extubation should include using a device as a guide for expedited reintubation.[1] Stylets and intubating bougies have a hollow core and can be used as a temporary means of oxygenation and ventilation.[1] Difficult extubation is rare and occurs in cases such as unknown subglottic stenosis, severe edema, or surgical related factor such as the endotracheal tube (ETT) being anchored to the tracheal wall. Airway obstruction is the main cause of extubation failure and need for reintubation after anesthesia. Factors are patient-related, surgery-related, and provider-related such as inappropriate or incomplete planning, management, judgment.[12,13]

Weaning Failure

Weaning failure relates to the necessity of ventilator support and intolerance of spontaneous respiration without it. Treatment consists of reintubation, invasive ventilation, and noninvasive ventilation in some patients. Both tend to occur within 72 hours of extubation. In the postoperative setting and in the intensive care unit (ICU), extubation failure most commonly occurs within 2 hours after removing the endotracheal tube. This should be considered when deciding the length of time in which to maintain airway exchange catheters in place as well as to monitor patients at risk of extubation failure (**Table 3**).[12]

Table 3 Conditions associated with increased risk of extubation failure	
Obesity and obstructive sleep apnea	OSA patient undergoing surgery for OSA treatment has as high as 5% incidence of postoperative airway complications[12]
Major head, neck, or upper airway surgery	Reintubation rates of 0.7%–11.1%; neck radiation changes most significant clinical predictor of impossible mask ventilation, extreme neck rigidity, modification of normal airway anatomy with significant tracheal intubation difficulty and impossible emergency tracheostomy, postradiation edema, impair lymphatic drainage after neck dissection
Obstetric procedures	Airway edema and obesity
Cervical spine procedures	Anterior cervical spine (cspine) surgery risk of airway compromise immediately and for up to 48 h after procedure, retropharyngeal hematoma Risks: surgery >5 h, >3 vertebral levels that include c2 c3 or c4, ebl above 300. Requires close respiratory monitoring of the patients for 48 h

Abbreviation: ebl, estimated blood loss.
Data from Cavallone LF, Vannucci A. Review article: extubation of the difficult airway and extubation failure. Anesth Analg 2013;116(2):368–83.

Extubation-Related Airway Complications or Airway-Related Adverse Events at Extubation

Extubation failure relates to the inability to maintain the airway upon removal of the endotracheal tube, and reintubation is usually the treatment. Causes are most often due to airway obstruction such as:

- Laryngeal obstruction: swelling after multiple intubation attempts, upper airway and major neck surgery, airway trauma and burns, prone or Trendelenburg positioning, hypervolemia, prolonged tracheal intubation, long-term effects of radiation, accumulation of secretions. Laryngeal edema is the most frequent cause of obstruction in early extubation failure in both ICU and postoperative patients.[12]
- Laryngospasm: contraction of adductor muscles of vocal cords causing complete glottic obstruction. Use of LMAs in adults can reduce this, but risk increases in children, particularly following upper respiratory infections. The major associated complication is negative pressure pulmonary edema, especially in young healthy male patients, which may lead to tracheobronchial and alveolar hemorrhage.
- Vocal cord paralysis due to recurrent laryngeal nerve injury: this most commonly occurs following thyroid surgery but has also been associated with cervical and intrathoracic procedures. Unilateral injury is normally asymptomatic, but bilateral injury results in immediate obstruction with stridor.
- Postoperative bleeding can cause external compression due to hematoma or internal obstruction due to clots.
- Collapse of the airway: upper airway soft tissue collapse due to anesthetics, opioids, and muscle relaxants. Tracheomalacia can cause tracheal collapse.

In the ICU, the reintubation incidence is 0.4% to 25% in critically ill patients and has direct correlation between prolonged ICU and hospital stay and mortality. Weaning failure has higher mortality (30%–52.9%) than airway obstruction (7%–17.4%).[14] Unplanned extubation occurs in 5% to 15% of ICU intubated patients and is associated with increased ICU morbidity[15] and mortality.

FOLLOW-UP CARE

Although there are no set guidelines or sufficient evidence for follow-up care regarding a patient who presented with a difficult airway, several recommendations are in place for patient safety:

1. Documentation of airway management
2. Informing and advising the patient or responsible person of the occurrence and potential life-threatening complications associated with difficult airway in order to facilitate delivery of future care
3. Documentation of presence and nature of difficult airway, description of difficulties with facemask or supraglottic airway, or tracheal intubation. Description of techniques used and the extent in which they helped or were detrimental.
4. A notification bracelet, chart flag, or letter should be provided to the patient.[1,2]

SUMMARY

Airway management skills are critical to patient care in many settings. Patients with a difficult airway present unique challenges and considerations. It is recommended that clinicians assess patients for a possible difficult airway by obtaining a thorough history and physical examination. Familiarity with difficult airway management guidelines, algorithms, tools, and techniques is essential to formulating a safe and effective plan for intubation as well as extubation of patients with this condition.

REFERENCES

1. Apfelbaum JL, Hagberg CA, Caplan RA, et al. Practice guidelines for management of the difficult airway: an updated report by the American Society of Anesthesiologists Task Force on management of the difficult airway. Anesthesiology 2013;118(2):251–70.
2. Rosenblatt WH, Sukhupragarn W. Airway management. In: Barash PG, Cullen BF, Stoelting R, et al, editors. Clinical anesthesia. 7th edition. Philadelphia, PA: Lippincott Williams & Wilkins; 2014. p. 762–802.
3. Rosenblatt WH. The airway approach algorithm: a decision tree for organizing preoperative airway information. J Clin Anesth 2004;16(4):312–6.
4. Prevention CfDCa. Disability and obesity. 2014. Available at: http://www.cdc.gov/ncbddd/disabilityandhealth/obesity.html. Accessed August 27, 2014.
5. Gupta S, Sharma R, Jain D. Airway assessment: predictors of difficult airway. Indian J Anaesth 2005;49(4):257–62.
6. Ovassapian A, Glassenberg R, Randel GI, et al. The unexpected difficult airway and lingual tonsil hyperplasia: a case series and a review of the literature. Anesthesiology 2002;97(1):124–32.
7. Mallampati S. Clinical assessment of airway. Anesthesiol Clin North America 1995;13(2):301–6.
8. Shippey B, Ray D, McKeown D. Case series: the McGrath videolaryngoscope—an initial clinical evaluation. Can J Anaesth 2007;54(4):307–13.
9. Rosenstock CV, Thogersen B, Afshari A, et al. Awake fiberoptic or awake video laryngoscopic tracheal intubation in patients with anticipated difficult airway management: a randomized clinical trial. Anesthesiology 2012;116(6):1210–6.
10. Hagberg CA, Vartazarian TN, Chelly JE, et al. The incidence of gastroesophageal reflux and tracheal aspiration detected with pH electrodes is similar with the Laryngeal Mask Airway and Esophageal Tracheal Combitube—a pilot study. Can J Anaesth 2004;51(3):243–9.
11. Hagberg C. Current concepts in the management of the difficult airway. Anesthesiology News 2013;29(1):135–46.
12. Cavallone LF, Vannucci A. Review article: extubation of the difficult airway and extubation failure. Anesth Analg 2013;116(2):368–83.
13. American Society of Anesthesiologists Task Force on Management of the Difficult Airway. Practice guidelines for management of the difficult airway: an updated report by the American Society of Anesthesiologists Task Force on Management of the Difficult Airway. Anesthesiology 2003;98(5):1269–77.
14. Mort TC. Continuous airway access for the difficult extubation: the efficacy of the airway exchange catheter. Anesth Analg 2007;105(5):1357–62 [table of contents].
15. Thille AW, Harrois A, Schortgen F, et al. Outcomes of extubation failure in medical intensive care unit patients. Crit Care Med 2011;39(12):2612–8.

Intraoperative Fluid Management

Judy Thompson, CRNA, DNAP, APRN

KEYWORDS

- Body fluid compartments • Fluid management • Crystalloids and colloids
- Blood and blood products • The third space • Goal-directed fluid therapy

KEY POINTS

- The amount of fluid in an average adult is approximately 60% of their total body weight.
- The "4-2-1 Rule" is still used as a formula that gives a basic number for calculating requirements for fluid maintenance.
- Newer nil per os guidelines developed in 1999 should be used when calculating a fluid deficit.
- Data from randomized controlled trials do not support resuscitation with colloids (compared with crystalloids) as being associated with lower mortality.
- "The Third Space" is now deemed "a myth."
- Goal-directed fluid therapy is the current best practice recommendation for the management of high-acuity patients and/or complex or prolonged surgical procedures.

INTRODUCTION

A core element in the practice of anesthesia is the administration of intravenous (IV) fluids to maintain homeostasis. Clinical outcome data and evidence-based medicine direct best practice. Knowledge and understanding of the effects of fluid management choices should guide the clinical management of all patients and all procedures. The appropriate administration of IV fluids and blood products is equal in importance to the maintenance of sleep, the relief of pain, surgical muscle relaxation, and the monitoring of vital signs. This article explores currently available IV fluids, discusses current recommendations for their use, and cites recent studies that challenge some of the long established tenets of intraoperative fluid therapy. Goal-directed fluid therapy for select patients has been frequently studied and highly supported in the recent literature. This supportive evidence is examined, the monitoring modalities used and recommended criteria for patient and case selection are explained, and anticipated outcomes are

Disclosure Statement: The author has nothing to disclose.
Nurse Anesthesia Program, School of Nursing, Quinnipiac University, 275 Mount Carmel Avenue NH-HSC, Hamden, CT 06518, USA
E-mail address: judy.thompson@quinnipiac.edu

Crit Care Nurs Clin N Am 27 (2015) 67–77
http://dx.doi.org/10.1016/j.cnc.2014.10.012   ccnursing.theclinics.com

defined. Current evidence-supported recommendations for colloid and blood administration are also reviewed.

BODY FLUID COMPARTMENTS

Before intraoperative fluid management and replacement can be completely understood, it is important to review body fluid compartments, fluid distribution, and fluid composition. The body is in large part composed of fluid, ranging between 46% and 80%, depending on the age and gender of the individual and the body's composition of fat relative to muscle.[1(p382)] Pound for pound (or kilogram for kilogram), fat contains less fluid than muscle. Infants have the greatest percentage of total body fluid (70%–80% of their body weight), whereas the elderly have the least (50% of their body weight). Using an average amount of fluid at approximately 60% of the body weight, the hypothetical 70-kg (154-lb) adult (if one were to lose all of their bodily fluid) would weigh 42 kg (61.6 lb). As you can see, we are mostly water. The other tissues are "light weights" compared with total body water (TBW).

TBW is divided between 2 compartments within the body, the intracellular (ICF) and extracellular (ECF) fluids. The intracellular compartment contains most of the body water, comprising about two-thirds of the total fluid volume. The ECF compartment therefore contains the other one-third of the total fluid volume. The ECF compartment is further divided into the intravascular fluid (ICF or plasma) that makes up approximately one-quarter of the ECF and the interstitial fluid (ISF) that makes up the rest. ICF is high in potassium and magnesium and low in sodium and chloride ions. The ECF composition is the opposite of that of the ICF, low in potassium and magnesium and high in sodium and chloride ions.

Semipermeable cell and capillary membranes separate the fluid compartments. The ICF compartment is separated from the ECF compartment by a cell membrane, and the ICF is separated from the ISF by a capillary membrane. The properties of the membrane that separates the fluid compartment as well as the relative concentration of the osmotically active substances within each compartment are the factors primarily responsible for the movement of fluid (water and electrolytes) among compartments in the body.[1(p382)] This movement is governed by Starling forces. Starling forces maintain the balance between hydrostatic pressure of the blood in the capillaries and the osmotic attraction of the blood for the surrounding fluid. Starling forces are made up of ISF pressure, ISF colloid osmotic pressure, capillary pressure, and plasma colloid osmotic pressures, respectively.[2]

Preoperatively, one can attempt to assess the fluid status of patients by several indices, such as skin turgor, mucus membrane hydration, heart rate, blood pressure and pulses, urinary output, and laboratory findings, such as specific gravity and osmolality of the urine, serial hematocrit (HCT), blood urea nitrogen (BUN), creatinine, and BUN/creatinine ratio, serum sodium, arterial blood gases, and base deficits. All of these measures are indirect indices. None of them in isolation or together are definitive. If the patient was known to have had vomiting and/or diarrhea preoperatively or a fever, or had been actively bleeding before surgery, this deficit could be attempted to be calculated as well and a plan devised for fluid replacement and maintenance therapy. Again, this is not definitive and in certain circumstances may be all that there is to use as a guide. At the time anesthesia is induced and throughout the intraoperative period, yet another set of variables exist that can be used to measure directly, such as response to anesthetics, pulses, and urinary output if a Foley catheter is in place. In addition to urinary output, blood and fluid loss can be estimated by measuring suction from the surgical site or from oral/

nasogastric tube drainage, chest tube drainage, sponges, and gauzes (depending on their level of saturation).

FLUID COMPOSITION

IV fluids may be broadly classified into colloid and crystalloid solutions. They each have very different physical, chemical, and physiologic characteristics. Crystalloids are solutions of inorganic ions and small organic molecules dissolved in water. They are the most common fluids administered intraoperatively to patients. Infused crystalloids are free of colloid osmotic force and are therefore not retained at the vascular wall. Accordingly, they distribute within the whole extracellular space for physiologic reasons.[3]

Crystalloids have as wide a range of uses as they have compositions (**Table 1**). The main solute is either glucose or sodium chloride (saline) and the solutions may be isotonic, hypotonic, or hypertonic with respect to plasma.[4] Crystalloids that most closely compare to the composition of plasma are also referred to as "balanced." When glucose is added to an isotonic solution, it is quickly metabolized, which allows the water in the solution to be freely distributed throughout the TBW. For this reason, the addition of glucose to a crystalloid provides water replacement and is used to treat simple dehydration. The most common balanced salt solutions used during surgery are 0.9% sodium chloride (normal saline, NS) and lactated Ringer's solution (LR). Isotonic solutions such as NS and LR are commonly used to correct the hypovolemia resulting from surgery and anesthesia because the bulk of fluid lost is isotonic.[1(p392)] Crystalloids have an intravascular half-life of approximately 20 to 30 minutes.

Colloids are large molecular weight solutions that do not easily pass the endothelial wall.[5] Colloid molecules are most commonly dissolved in isotonic saline, but they may also be dissolved in isotonic glucose, hypertonic saline, and isotonic "balanced" electrolyte solutions. Colloids expand plasma volume by 1:1. Colloid solutions are divided into semisynthetic and naturally occurring human plasma derivatives. Blood derivatives include fresh frozen plasma (FFP) and plasma protein fraction (PPF) and albumin. Albumin comes in 5% and 25% solutions and is purified from human plasma. The half-life in human plasma is approximately 16 hours. PPF comes in a 5% solution and contains α-globulins and β-globulins plus albumin. These blood derivatives are heated to 60°C for 10 minutes to minimize the risk of transmitting hepatitis and other virally transmitted diseases as well as bacterial contamination.

Table 1
Commonly used crystalloids

Solution	Tonicity	Na$^+$	Cl$^-$	K$^+$	Ca^{++}	Glucose	Lactate
			Fluid Management				
D5W	Hypo					50	
NS	Iso	154	154				
D51/4 NS	Iso	38.5	38.5			50	
D51/2 NS	Hyper	77	77			50	
D5NS	Hyper	154	154			50	
LR	Iso	130	109	4	3		28
PL	Iso	140	98	5			
D5LR	Hyper	130	109	4	3	50	28
½ NS	Hypo	77	77				

Semisynthetic colloids include gelatins, dextrans, and hydroxyethyl starches. Dextran is a polysaccharide made of many glucose molecules. Dextran 70 (Macrodex) is the most widely used plasma expander, which yields the same volume as the infused amount or a 1:1 ratio. The solution resides in the plasma for about 3 to 4 hours.[6] Dextran 40 (Rheomacrodex) is used in vascular surgery because it decreases blood viscosity and improves blood flow through the microcirculation. These synthetic products are not without several associated problems. They have been implicated in both anaphylactic and anaphylactoid reactions. The administration of a low-molecular-weight dextran (dextran-1 Promit, Hapten) before starting the infusion can considerably reduce the possibility of these serious reactions. Dextran can interfere with blood typing, can prolong bleeding time, can exhibit antiplatelet effects, and has been associated with renal failure as well. The alterations in platelet function, thus increasing the potential for blood loss, are the basis for the maximum dose recommendations of 1.5 to 2 g/kg for such solutions.[7]

Hydroxyethyl starch (Hetastarch) is a 6% solution. The molecules are smaller and therefore more easily eliminated by the kidneys. Hetastarch is a highly effective plasma expander, is less expensive than albumin, is nonantigenic, and does not affect bleeding times and coagulation to the extent that the dextrans do.

Much controversy regarding the use of crystalloids versus colloids has been present in recent literature. According to an analysis of the literature in the Cochrane Database, "there is no evidence from randomized controlled trials that resuscitation with colloids reduces the risk of death, compared to resuscitation with crystalloids, in patients with trauma, burns or following surgery. Furthermore, the use of hydroxyethyl starch might increase mortality. As colloids are not associated with an improvement in survival and are considerably more expensive than crystalloids, it is hard to see how their continued use in clinical practice can be justified."[8]

THE CALCULATION OF FLUID MAINTENANCE

The calculation of maintenance fluid requirements is of particular use in the estimation of electrolyte and water deficits in preoperative surgical patients. Commonly, these patients have been restricted from eating and drinking for a prolonged period of time. In healthy adults, sufficient water is required to balance gastrointestinal losses of 100 to 200 mL/d, insensible losses of 500 to 1000 mL/d (half of which is respiratory and half is cutaneous), and urinary losses of 1000 mL/d.[9]

It might be hard to believe, but the widely used formula for calculating fluid maintenance requirements came from the work of Holliday and Segar[10] in 1957. In their publication, they advocated for the use of hourly fluid maintenance based on caloric expenditure calculated by weight (**Fig. 1**). Their work was directed at the pediatric patient initially. Anesthesia providers have widely used this formula in their calculation of intraoperative fluid maintenance. This commonly used formula is the "4-2-1 Rule," which has been the basis for fluid calculations since its adoption (**Fig. 1**). Holliday and Segar formulated this simple rule from the following:

Hourly volume (V1) = Maintenance (M) + Fasting deficit (nil per os [NPO]) + Estimated Blood Loss (EBL) + Third Space Losses (TS).[11]

The practitioners has used the "4-2-1 Rule" in practice, taught it to new practitioners, and relied on it to give initial calculations for many years. This equation has been the basis from which many additional fluid calculations have been derived. A simple example follows.

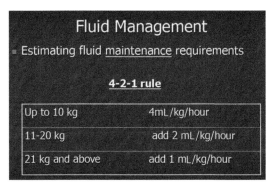

Fig. 1. Commonly used formula for fluid maintenance requirements (Holliday and Segar) "4-2-1 Rule." (*Data from* Holliday MA, Segar WE. The maintenance need for water in parenteral fluid therapy. Pediatrics 1957;19(5):823–32.)

- The hypothetical 70-kg adult: 4 mL per kilogram for the first 10 kg (40 mL), 2 mL for the next 10 kg (20 mL), and 1 mL for each kilogram greater than 21 kg (50 mL) = 40 + 20 + 50 = 110 mL/h for maintenance.

Eighteen years later, expanded recommendations were published that became widely adopted as well.[12] These recommendations were used to correct for the NPO deficit, which was commonly calculated from midnight to the time of surgery (at least 8 hours after fast) the following day. Although the current recommendations published in 1999 do not support these past NPO guidelines,[13] this practice is still commonly used in many settings (**Table 2**).

If calculations are based on the "4-2-1 Rule" and the NPO deficit is added for each hour that the patient has fasted (liquid and solid), the result will be roughly this formula: Maintenance × Hours fasted = Deficit.

- The hypothetical patient of 70 kg: Maintenance (110 mL) × 8 hours = 880 (fluid deficit).

Replacing this has been traditionally broken into set amounts and added to the hourly maintenance. The most commonly used method by clinicians is to divide this

Table 2
Current NPO guidelines

The NPO Requirement	
Clear liquids	2 h
Breast milk	4 h
Formula/milk	6 h
Light meal (clear liquid/toast)	6 h
Solid food	8 h

Guidelines prefer relatively health patients without risk factors for delayed gastric emptying. Patients undergoing emergency surgery or patients with predisposing factors for delayed gastric emptying (diabetics, morbidly obese, pregnant, gastroesophageal reflux disease, difficult airway) should follow the NPO guidelines (nothing by mouth for 8 h).
    Data from Practice guidelines for preoperative fasting and the use of pharmacologic agents to reduce the risk of pulmonary aspiration: application to healthy patients undergoing elective procedures: a report by the American Society of Anesthesiologists Task Force on Preoperative Fasting. Anesthesiology 1999;90(3):896–905.

amount by 1/2 and give it back to the patient in the first hour of surgery. This amount, of course, is plus the maintenance. The second hour, one-quarter of the deficit plus the maintenance is replaced, and in the third hour, the final one-quarter of the deficit is replaced, making the calculated total, which would look like this:

- 110 mL (calculated maintenance) + 880 (calculated deficit)/2 or 440 mL = 550 mL (total) given in the first hour.
- 110 mL (maintenance) + (880/4) 220 mL (1/4 of the calculated deficit) = 330 mL for the second hour.
- 110 mL + (880/4) (=220) = 330 for the third hour.

Therefore, in 3 hours, the patient would receive a total of (550 mL + 330 mL + 330 mL) or 1210 mL of fluid. This amount, provided all variables stay the same, should replace the patient's deficit from fasting.

If the fast were to follow the newer guidelines, only an 8-hour deficit would be seen in a patient with solid food intake preoperatively or in a patient with certain comorbidities (see **Table 2**). In other patients, the current NPO guidelines would be followed and the hours actually fasted used to calculate the deficit. This amount might be a deficit that is so insignificant that it is not realty worth including in the calculations.

In this example, a toddler coming for surgery nursed 4 hours previously.

- Example: 13-kg toddler, NPO for 4 hours
  - 46 mL × 4 hours = 184 mL (deficit)
  - 1st hour, 92 mL + 46 = 138 mL (138 mL)
  - 2nd hour, 46 mL + 46 mL = 92 mL (230 mL)
  - 3rd hour, 46 mL + 46 mL = 92 mL (322 mL)

THE THIRD SPACE

Until recently, calculating surgical fluid replacement was normally based on 4 parameter: maintenance, deficits, surgical wound losses, and "third space" losses. The notion of a "third space" was originally postulated by Shires and colleagues[14] in 1961 around the time of the Vietnam Conflict when mass casualties were being treated in the field. The third space, according to Shires, consisted of fluid that was sequestered into a compartment that was no longer functional due most often to tissue trauma. Examples of a "third space" might be ascites or fluid in the peritoneal cavity or bowel or from traumatized tissues. In the past, these calculations were added to the fluids that were transfused into the patients, depending on an estimation of the degree of trauma produced by a particular procedure. **Table 3** gives an example of these calculations. If the surgery caused minimal tissue trauma such as one might expect from a small incision such as an appendectomy, an additional fluid requirement of between 1 and 4 mL/kg/h would be added to the maintenance for each hour of surgery. Larger

Table 3
The hypothetical "third space" requirements

Fluid Management	
Degree of Tissue Trauma	Additional Fluid Requirement
Minimal (eg, herniorrhaphy)	0–4 mL/kg/h
Moderate (eg, cholecystectomy)	4–6 mL/kg/h
Severe (eg, bowel resection)	6–8 mL/kg/h

procedures that were more invasive and caused more severe tissue trauma required larger fluid requirements of as much as 8 mL/kg/h of surgery. Classic third space fluid losses have never been measured directly, and the actual location of the lost fluid remains unclear.[15] It is now known that the shift of fluid to the interstitial space is returned to the circulation via the lymphatics and is thus not lost to the circulation at all. Such shifting is related to a destruction of the endothelial glycocalyx, a key structure of the vascular barrier, by traumatic inflammation and iatrogenic hypervolemia.[3] The glycocalyx is the inner lining of the endothelial wall visible through electron microscopy. It consists of a variety of transmembrane and membrane-bound molecules. The glycocalyx is approximately 1 μm in thickness. Surgical stress is responsible for causing the release of several inflammatory mediators, atrial natriuretic peptide (ANP) among them. ANP release is triggered by acute hypervolemia that is often induced by iatrogenic administration of IV fluids. A degradation of the glycocalyx leads inevitably to an increase of capillary leakage and interstitial edema, which is strongly corelated to a decrease in tissue oxygenation.[16] Recent evidence now recommends that the arbitrary third space is no longer included in fluid calculations.

GOAL-DIRECTED FLUID THERAPY

Multiple studies done within the last 20 years have looked at fluid therapy based on a balance between inadequate fluid resuscitation and decreased tissue perfusion and excess fluid with edema formation. These studies have been casting doubt on the traditional management of fluid in favor of a more individualized fluid therapy based not only on the types of surgery but also on the individual characteristics of the patients. Studies have shown that patients undergoing major procedures can gain an average of between 3 and 10 kg of weight due to traditional methods of fluid therapy.[17] Tissue edema has been associated with altered oxygen tensions, and this directly affects surgical wound healing. Other studies have shown that mortality is higher in patients with further weight increases.[18] With the benefits of more sophisticated technology, fluid therapy may be more easily individualized today than ever before and is the basis for individualized fluid therapy, or goal-directed fluid therapy. Goal-directed fluid therapy is based on a specific endpoint.

One of the hallmark studies in fluid therapy and administration techniques was the study done by Brandstrup and colleagues[19] in 2003. Standard fluid therapy versus restricted fluid replacement was compared in patients undergoing colorectal surgery. In this study, researchers looked at 141 patients in 8 hospital trials. The findings indicated that patients in the restrictive group had a significantly lower incidence of cardiac and wound-healing complications compared with the patients in the standard group.

Technologies used to predict fluid responsiveness and to guide management for goal-directed fluid therapy in the intraoperative setting are not readily available in all settings and are costly to obtain. Esophageal Doppler monitoring is a minimally invasive method using ultrasound technology to assess the blood flow in the descending aorta, thereby guiding goal-directed fluid therapy in the operating room. A disposable probe is placed in the esophagus following induction of anesthesia.

The use of pulmonary artery catheters to assess fluid status has declined significantly because of inconsistencies in the data obtained and the complication rate associated with their use. Arterial pulse waveforms, while also invasive, can be used to predict fluid responsiveness through the measurement of pulse contour and pulse power analysis. The lithium dilution CO monitor and transesophageal echocardiography have been successfully used to guide goal-directed fluid therapy as well. Newer monitors available measure plethysmographic variability in both the pulse oximeter and the arterial waveforms and produce a plethysmographic variability index (PVI). Studies have shown this measurement to be reliant in patients in normal sinus rhythm and mechanically ventilated with tidal volumes and a heart rate to respiratory rate ratio within an acceptable range.[7] Monitors are commercially available that measure PVI among other parameters. This technology may become routine in the future and more readily available. Using new technology with goal-directed fluid therapy allows one to more carefully and accurately maintain the fluid requirements throughout the surgical procedure for the sickest patients and for the most critical procedures.

BLOOD COMPONENT THERAPY

Volume replacement due to intraoperative blood loss initially can be achieved with both crystalloids and colloids. If blood loss due to hemorrhage is significant enough that the danger of anemia outweighs the risk of transfusion and/or a decreased oxygen-carrying capacity is present, then the administration of blood may be required. Traditional therapy suggests that crystalloid replacement for blood volume lost is in a 1:3 ratio (for every measurable amount of blood lost, 3 times the amount of crystalloid needs to be administered). This ratio is for volume replacement lost only and for initial and noncritical blood loss. For colloids, the ratio is 1:1.

Decisions to administer blood must take into account several factors including not only the amount of blood lost, the clinical condition of the patient, and the availability of the proper type of blood, but also, on occasion, factors that are unrelated to the clinical picture, such as religious beliefs. Estimation of blood loss, patient-specific blood volume, and calculation of allowable blood loss can be done before transfusion is considered. There are several formulas that allow a reasonable estimate. To do this, one must first be able to calculate the patient's estimated blood volume. **Table 4** list the average blood volumes for men, women, and children. When calculating a potential allowable blood loss, it might be prudent to consider monitoring for hemoglobin concentration using a point-of-care monitor or the laboratory if one is not available. Healthy patients with hemoglobin values greater than 10 g/dL rarely require transfusion and those with hemoglobin values less than 6 g/dL almost always require transfusion. In patients with intermediate hemoglobin concentrations of between 10 and 6 g/dL, the decision should be based on the patient and/or the procedure. One of

Table 4 Average blood volumes	
Blood Therapy	
Average blood volumes	
Age	**Blood volume**
Neonates	
Preemies	95 mL/kg
Full term	85 mL/kg
Infants	80 mL/kg
Adults	
Men	75 mL/kg
Women	65 mL/kg

Box 1
Example: allowable blood loss to a hematocrit of 30%

Blood therapy

Blood

   Calculation of blood loss for HCT to decrease to 30%

     EBV

     Estimate RCV at the preoperative HCT (ERCV$_{preop}$)

     Estimate RBCV at HCT of 30% (ERCV$_{30\%}$)

       Assuming that fluid volume is maintained

     Calculate the RCV lost when the HCT is 30

       RBCV $_{lost}$ = RBCV$_{preop}$ − RBCV$_{30\%}$

      Allowable blood loss = RBCV$_{lost}$ × 3

---

the formulas used for calculating allowable blood loss is found in **Box 1** with an example found in **Box 2**. The following more simplified formula may also be used:

$$\text{Maximal allowable blood loss (MABL)} = \text{Estimated blood volume (EBV)} \times \frac{(\text{Starting HCT} - \text{Target HCT})}{\text{Starting HCT}}$$ [1(p392)]

The major goal of the administration of red blood cells (RBCs) is to treat anemia and thus to increase O_2 carrying capacity. The use of packed RBCs is the most common form of transfusion therapy for the treatment of anemia. Packed RBCs are reconstituted with between 50 and 100 mL of 0.9% NaCl (NS). Glucose solutions should never be used because they can cause hemolysis of the red cell. LR contains calcium and may cause clotting of the cells to occur because of the preservative citrate phosphate dextrose-adenine in the blood. One unit of RBCs will increase the hemoglobin concentration by 1 g/dL and the hemocrit by 2% to 3% in adults. A transfusion of 10 mL/kg of RBCs will increase the hemoglobin concentration by 3 g/dL and the hemocrit by 10%.

The administration of blood is not without associated hazards. Bacterial contamination is rare because the blood supply is carefully screened and tested. The number 1

Box 2
Example of allowable blood loss/65-kg woman to a hematocrit of 30%

Blood therapy

Example

   A 65-kg woman has a preoperative HCT of 34%.

   How much blood loss will decrease her HCT to 30%?

     EBV = 65 mL/kg × 65 kg = 4225 mL

     RBCV$_{34\%}$ = 4225 × 34% = 1436.5 mL

     RBCV$_{30\%}$ = 4225 × 30% = 1267.5 mL

     Red cell loss at 30% = 1436.5–1267.5 = 169 mL

     Allowable blood loss = 3 × 169 = 507 mL

---

cause of transfusion-related fatalities is transfusion-related acute lung injury (TRALI). TRALI occurs approximately 6 hours following the transfusion of blood or FFP. It is characterized by dyspnea and arterial hypoxemia secondary to noncardiogenic pulmonary edema fluid with a high protein content.

Other associated complications include transfusion reactions, febrile, allergic, and hemolytic, which can cause injury to the kidneys as well as death.

SUMMARY

In the past, direct and indirect indices were used to determine the fluid status of patients. Calculating preoperative deficits and planning for intraoperative maintenance have not significantly changed for many years. In practice, the "4-2-1 Rule" is still partially relied on for guidance. More evidence-based literature now challenges practices. The "third space" and its inclusion in the calculations have been proven to be the source of hypervolemia in many surgical patients. Newer and more sophisticated monitoring modalities allow more precise guidance and are being used more commonly with the sicker patients. Not only is intraoperative fluid maintenance being challenged, but more questions are arising about the best uses of these fluids. New evidence comparing colloids with crystalloids is supporting the latter in volume expansion and safety.

Health care providers need to individualize fluid administration based on many factors. Staying current on the latest evidence is needed to guide them in this important goal in the future.

REFERENCES

1. Waters E, Nishinago A. Fluids, electrolytes and blood component therapy. In: Nagelhout J, Plaus KL, editors. Nurse anesthesia. 5th edition. St Louis (MO): Elsevier; 2014. p. 382–402.
2. Guyton AC, Hall JE. The microcirculation and the lymphatic system: capillary fluid exchange, interstitial fluid and lymph flow. In: Guyton AC, Hall JE, editors. Textbook of medical physiology. 12th edition. Philadelphia: Saunders; 2011. p. 177–90.
3. Jacob M, Chappell D, Rehm M. The "third space"–fact or fiction? Best Pract Res Clin Anaesthesiol 2009;23:145–57.
4. Grocott MP, Mythen MG. Perioperative fluid management and clinical outcomes in adults. Anesth Analg 2005;100:1093–106.
5. Hemmings HC Jr, Egan TD. Pharmacology and physiology for anesthesia, foundations and clinical application. Philadelphia: Elsevier/Saunders; 2013.
6. Svensen C, Haun RG. Volume kinetics of Ringers solution, dextran 70 and hypertonic saline in male volunteers. Anesthesiology 1997;87:204–12.
7. Gallagher K, Vacchiano C. Reexamining traditional intraoperative fluid administration: evolving views in the age of goal-directed therapy. AANA J 2014;82(2): 235–42.
8. Perel P, Roberts I. Colloids versus crystalloids for fluid resuscitation in critically ill patients. Cochrane Database Syst Rev 2013;(2):CD000567.
9. Barash PG, Cullen BF, Stoelting RK, et al, editors. Clinical anesthesia. 7th edition. Philadelphia: Lippincott Williams and Wilkins; 2013. p. 333–9.
10. Holliday MA, Segar WE. The maintenance need for water in parenteral fluid therapy. Pediatrics 1957;19(5):823–32.
11. Morgan GE, Mikhail MS, Murray MJ. Clinical anesthesiology. 4th edition. New York: Lange Medical Books/McGraw-Hill; 2006.

12. Furman FB. Intraoperative fluid therapy. Int Anesthesiol Clin 1975;13(3):133–47.
13. Practice guidelines for preoperative fasting and the use of pharmacologic agents to reduce the risk of pulmonary aspiration: application to healthy patients undergoing elective procedures: a report by the American Society of Anesthesiologist Task Force on Preoperative Fasting. Anesthesiology 1999;90(3):896–905.
14. Shires T, Williams J, Brown F. Acute change in extracellular fluids associated with major surgical procedures. Ann Surg 1961;154(5):803–10.
15. Brandstrup B. Fluid therapy for the surgical patient. Best Pract Res Clin Anaesthesiol 2006;20:265–83.
16. Rehm M, Bruegger D, Christ F, et al. Shedding of the endothelial glycocalyx in patients undergoing major vascular surgery with global and regional ischemia. Circulation 2007;116:1896–906.
17. Joshi GP. Intraoperative fluid restriction improves outcome after major elective gastrointestinal surgery. Anesth Analg 2005;101(2):601–5.
18. Lowell JA, Schifferdecker C, Driscoll DF, et al. Perioperative fluid overload is not a benign problem. Crit Care Med 1990;18(7):728–33.
19. Brandstrup B, Tonnesen H, Beier-Holgersen R, et al, Danish Study Group on Perioperative Fluid Therapy. Effects of intravenous fluid restriction on postoperative complications: comparison of two perioperative fluid regimens: a randomized assessor-blinded multicenter trial. Ann Surg 2003;238(5):641–8.

Infection Control in the Operating Room

Marianne S. Cosgrove, CRNA, DNAP, APRN

KEYWORDS

- Infection control • Surgical site infection (SSI) • Operating room
- Anesthesia provider • Hand hygiene

KEY POINTS

- Surgical site infections (SSIs) occur in 160,000 to 300,000 patients per year, at a rate of 2% to 5%.
- SSIs increase postoperative hospitalization stay and the likelihood of postoperative mortality by a factor of 2- to 11-fold.
- The estimated financial impact of SSIs on the health care system ranges from $3.5 to $45.0 billion annually.
- Anesthesia providers have the potential to increase the patient's risk for developing an SSI.
- The use of antibiotics, attention to patient normothermia, and sound hand hygiene have been shown to decrease the rate of postoperative SSI.

INTRODUCTION

The incidence of nosocomial infections, or hospital-acquired infections (HAIs), continues to increase, despite heightened awareness of the issue and attempts to limit its occurrence. In the United States, an estimated 722,000 HAIs occurred in 2011, with a resultant 9.6% mortality rate.[1] It has been proposed that between 4% and 10% of hospitalized patients in the United States will acquire a nosocomial infection, particularly after entry into operating room (OR) or intensive care environments.[1,2] Between 2011 and 2012, an estimated 53,700 of these HAIs were surgical site infections (SSIs).[1] SSIs are now considered to be the most common and costly HAI, adding approximately 7 to 11 days to the expected postsurgical hospital stay and increasing perioperative morbidity and mortality. The health care expenditures associated with the occurrence of SSIs are roughly projected to be between $3.5 and $45.0 billion annually.[3,4] Although the problem of SSIs seems to be rampant and gaining momentum, an estimated 40% to 60% of these infections may actually be preventable.[4]

Department of Anesthesiology, Yale-New Haven Hospital School of Nurse Anesthesia, Yale University, Yale Medical Group/Yale-New Haven Hospital – SRC, 1450 Chapel Street, New Haven, CT 06511, USA
E-mail address: marianne.cosgrove@yale.edu

Crit Care Nurs Clin N Am 27 (2015) 79–87
http://dx.doi.org/10.1016/j.cnc.2014.10.004
ccnursing.theclinics.com

Bearing these disconcerting facts in mind, it has been widely recognized that the OR milieu may be a key contributor to the development of HAIs, particularly with regard to SSIs. Although the genesis of these infections may be multifactorial, 2 key themes have emerged: (1) human-controlled vector transmission of pathogens, and (2) physical factors such as the presence of a multitude of surfaces in the OR setting which may be difficult to cleanse because of inherent texture or location. Areas such as those found on the anesthesia workstation may harbor considerable infective material, both visible and occult.[5–7] This fact is further compounded by the finding that anesthetist hand hygiene practices are largely inadequate.[2,6–9]

Overall, the hospital environment is a breeding ground for various types of bacteria, with a magnified effect in the intensive care units and the operating suites. In a study conducted in 2008 by Al-Hamad and Maxwell,[10] frequently touched surfaces found in the hospital setting were tested for the presence of resident microbial agents. Bed frames, telephones, and computer keyboards were among the items that yielded the highest total viable bacterial counts. Although the pathogen subtypes were varied, these cultures often included the dangerous methicillin-resistant *Staphylococcus aureus* (MRSA).[10–13]

After a systematic review of the current literature, and drawing from circumstantial experiences of this certified registered nurse anesthetist (CRNA) author within the OR setting, the issues listed in **Box 1** may increase the incidence of nosocomial infection emanating specifically from the perioperative period. **Fig. 1**, adapted from Thiele and colleagues,[23] aptly depicts the interface between infectious agents and their various vectors and routes to the patient in the operating room.

It follows reason that the frequent use of keyboards for electronic intraoperative charting by the anesthesia provider may further aggravate an already grim situation with respect to the escalating rate of nosocomial infection.[7,16,19] With the increasing use of electronic medical records (EMRs) in ORs nationwide, the latent risk of contamination of related equipment exists during the course of a procedure, with subsequent transmission to the patient.[2,7,11–13,19] Specifically, the anesthetist may contaminate the computer keyboard and mouse during use with gloved (or bare) hands while simultaneously administering patient care and documenting intraoperative events, through the inadvertent transfer of blood and pathogens from the patient to equipment. For example, contact with the patient's mouth occurs during intubation, transferring oral flora onto the provider's hands. Likewise, insertion of intravenous catheters or invasive monitors may cause soiling of the anesthetist's gloves with blood or related body fluids. Although the usual practice is to remove soiled gloves after each procedure and replace with a clean pair, this may not always occur. Because of the rapid pace of the induction sequence and the occasional need to respond quickly to untoward events during the course of other procedures, the CRNA, student registered nurse anesthetist, anesthesiologist, or resident may unknowingly transfer infective pathogens onto the anesthesia workstation and the EMR–human interface while wearing contaminated gloves. Furthermore, equipment contained in anesthesia cart drawers may be inadvertently contaminated if the anesthesia provider attempts to quickly retrieve items while wearing soiled gloves.

Disinfection of keyboards between patients is difficult because of the inherent multi-surfaced nature of these devices. Despite the presence of a washable vinyl or rubber covering that typically encapsulates the various computer keyboards found in the OR, significant microbial contamination with MRSA and variants may potentially be left behind, particularly in the spaces between keys, even after careful decontamination with bleach or alcohol-containing wipes.[2,11–14]

Box 1
Issues that may increase the incidence of nosocomial infection in the perioperative period

Anesthetist factors

- Colonization with microbiome[2,6,10]
- Poor hand washing techniques/habits before procedures, at the beginning of the procedures, and between patient contact[2,7,9]
- Contact with previously contaminated surfaces, with subsequent transmission to patients[14]
- Presence of jewelry; use of artificial nails
- Wearing scrubs home; entering hospital wearing home-laundered scrubs
- Sequestration at the head of the bed; low visibility of actions to other OR staff[2]
- Performance of procedures without use of gloves (eg, suctioning, intravenous starts, emptying of urinary catheter)
- Increased task density coupled with the need to respond quickly to abrupt changes in patient condition
- The presence of production pressure leading to rushing
- Inadequate cleaning of monitoring equipment/anesthesia workstation between patients
- Failure to administer preincision antibiotics in a timely manner[15–17]
- Gender: women have higher bacterial counts; men are less apt to practice hand hygiene
- Failure to practice/maintain sound sterile technique when performing invasive procedures
- Reuse of items that have potentially been contaminated (eg, picking up items from the floor)
- Personal items brought into OR[18]
- Repeated use of uncovered intravenous stopcocks[2,7,9]
- Use of multidose vials without alcohol preparation or that may have expired
- Syringe and/or needle reuse between patients ("a never event")
- Use of electronic medical record equipment, such as computer mouse and keyboard, with soiled bare or gloved hands[2,7,9,11–13,16,19]

Patient factors

- Colonization with microbiome[2,20]
- Colonization with resistant/opportunistic bacterial strains (eg, MRSA, vancomycin-resistant enterococci), with subsequent contamination of surfaces[14]
- Presence of biofilms on patient transferred to OR surfaces[2,20]
- Comorbidities that increase the likelihood of infection/sepsis (eg, immunosuppression, chronic renal failure, diabetes mellitus)
- Active infectious disease
- Suppression of the immune response from administration of general anesthesia[2]
- Hypothermia[21]

OR environment

- Increased foot traffic in and out during procedures[22]
- Inattention to proper sterile technique
- Poor air flow/quality[23]
- OR design that facilitates spread of pathogens[23]
- Multiple surfaces/textures that may harbor bacteria

- Aerosolization of body fluids, particularly when power tools are used
- Occult contamination of monitoring equipment and/or surfaces[5]
- Improper/inadequate cleaning techniques between cases
- Presence of biofilms on OR surfaces[20]
- Ubiquitous use of tape on anesthesia equipment (machine, intravenous poles), which leaves tacky residue to which pathogens can adhere

Because of the congested and often disorganized nature of the anesthesia workstation,[24] the keyboard and the crevice-laden mouse will likely be contaminated multiple times during the course of anesthesia administration. This contamination occurs partly from the deposition of used syringes and airway equipment in proximity to or direct contact with these instruments, and the inadvertent use of the equipment with bare or soiled, gloved hands.

As demonstrated by Joga and Palumbo[25] in 2012, the combination of using hand sanitizer before making contact with the computer system and using disinfecting wipes to clean the system after contact may be effective in reducing the number of pathogens found at the computer site. Even though the investigators were able to successfully eliminate coliform bacteria on the surfaces of the computer systems, coagulase positive staphylococci were still detected, even after decontamination.

In addition, most EMR systems feature computer touchscreens, which may also be decontaminated between cases using only water as the cleansing agent. Although water is not effective in sanitizing these monitor touchscreens (and may actually facilitate hand-to-patient transmission of bioinfective material), bactericidal agents such as bleach may leave a residue, ultimately impeding visualization of the monitor display and eventually damaging the touchscreen. Therefore, it is hypothesized that these essential components of EMR systems may also constitute a fomite-like source of contamination between patients and may contribute profoundly to the staggering rate of perioperative infection.

Although the application of various modalities for the prevention of SSIs have been advocated, such as preoperative and postoperative supplemental oxygen administration, prophylactic use of intranasal mupirocin ointment, and tight perioperative glucose control, it has been suggested that attention to 3 specific interventions may help assuage the precipitous increase in the occurrence of nosocomial infections:

- Strict attention to hand hygiene
- Maintenance of patient normothermia
- Administration of preincision or procedure antibiotics with redosing at prescribed intervals

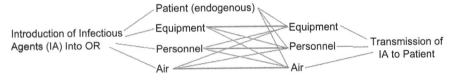

Fig. 1. Potential modes of transmission of IA to the surgical patient. (*From* Thiele RH, Huffmyer JL, Nemergut EC. The "six sigma" approach to the operating room environment and infection. Best Pract Res Clin Anaesthesiol 2008;22(3):538; with permission.)

Hand Hygiene

Of the 3 interventions noted to be most efficacious in preventing nosocomial infection, the most elemental is proper hand hygiene. Despite the simplistic nature of the act of hand washing and sanitizing with antiseptic gels, external forces such as production pressure, sequestration in the OR with limited access to wash stations, potential for skin irritation with antiseptic scrubs, and the lack of hand sanitization stations may impede the anesthetist from performing this most basic, albeit crucial task.

Human hands are well-known to harbor a multitude of bacterial flora, both resident and transient. However, because of repeated exposures to pathogenic bacteria, health care workers are at increased risk for persistent colonization with pathogens such as gram-negative bacilli, S aureus, and yeast. These pathogens may be transmitted easily to patients, particularly in the absence of sound hand hygiene practices.[26] In 2011, Loftus and colleagues[9] sampled the hands of anesthesia providers before the start of intraoperative care. They found that approximately 66% of provider hands were contaminated with at least 1 major pathogen, including MRSA, vancomycin-resistant enterococci, Enterococcus, methicillin-sensitive S aureus, and Enterobacteriaceae. In a controversial study undertaken by Biddle and Shah[6] in 2013, hand washing practices of anesthesia providers were monitored by clandestine observers in a large metropolitan OR. The researchers' intent was to quantify hand hygiene behaviors and to delineate the root causes of the failure to execute these practices. The results were staggering. After approximately 8000 observed opportunities for hand washing, anesthesia providers failed to perform this practice at an estimated rate of 82%. The authors suggested that these departures from normal protocol may have been from factors such as high task density and rushing secondary to widespread production pressure. Despite the fact that extenuating circumstances surround the anesthetic care of patients, anesthetists should ensure that hand washing always occurs at the following junctures:

- Before and after patient contact
- Before gloving to perform sterile procedures
- After performing invasive or "dirty" procedures, once gloves are removed
- Between patient contact

In addition, although a lack of evidence supports the diminution of SSIs after the removal of jewelry and nail polish,[4] common sense would dictate that the wearing of jewelry be kept to a minimum and nails be trimmed and clean, even in the presence of gloving.

Intraoperative Temperature Regulation

The presence of intraoperative hypothermia may precipitate a cascade of events that place the surgical patient at risk for the development of an SSI. In response to a reduction in core body temperature, physiologic activities such as vasoconstriction, suppression of phagocytic activity, decreased neutrophil activity, and diminished oxidative killing of bacteria may all contribute to the eventual development of an SSI.[9] In addition, once a patient becomes hypothermic, restoration of normal core body temperature may take hours to achieve, and persistent decreased core temperature may extend well into the postoperative period. Heat loss occurs through the following mechanisms: radiation (40%), convection and evaporation (30%), and conduction (30%). Other physiologic derangements noted with the institution of hypothermia are listed in **Box 2**.

Box 2
Physiologic derangements noted with the institution of hypothermia

- Vasoconstriction/increased systemic vascular resistance
- Shivering
- Increased oxygen consumption
- Increased myocardial work
- Prolonged bleeding time
- Delayed drug metabolism
- Arrhythmias
- Leftward shift of the oxygen–hemoglobin dissociation curve

Additionally, temperature regulation is a difficult issue to contend with because of a variety of intraoperative factors that may promote hypothermia (**Box 3**).

Intraoperative hypothermia occurs in 3 distinct phases:

1. Redistribution of heat from the core to the periphery secondary to vasodilation (first hour of surgery; 1°–2° decline)
2. Steady decline (over the next 2–4 hours) from radiant loss to the environment
3. Equilibration, where heat loss equals metabolic rate[27]

It is widely accepted that the most efficacious intervention to maintain core body temperature is via prewarming (before entry into the OR suite) and use of forced-air heaters during surgery.[21,23] Other recommended modalities for maintaining normothermia are as follows:

- Maintenance of ambient temperature in the OR
- Use of a fluid warmer
- Use of a respiratory heat and moisture exchanger (eg, Humid-Vent)
- Application of head and foot covering
- Institution of warming in the postoperative area[21]

Box 3
Intraoperative factors that contribute to hypothermia

- Decreased ambient temperature in the OR
- Patient anxiety
- Extreme age
- Patient comorbidity (eg, peripheral vascular disease)
- Patient exposure
- Application of wet preparation solutions
- Institution of general anesthesia (secondary to vasodilation)
- Institution of regional anesthesia (secondary to vasodilation)
- Infusion of room-temperature fluids at a rapid rate
- Decreased metabolic activity under general anesthesia
- Administration of anesthetic using high flows from the machine

---

Table 1
Guidelines for antimicrobial prophylaxis for surgery

Antimicrobial Agent	Recommended Dose (IV)	Redosing Interval
Cefazolin	2 g (3 g if pt wt >120 kg) 30 mg/kg (pediatric)	q3–4h
Cefotetan	2 g	q6h
Cefoxitin	2 g	q2h
Ciprofloxacin	400 mg	N/A
Metronidazole	500 mg	N/A
Vancomycin	1 g (15 mg/kg)	N/A
Gentamicin	80 mg (5 mg/kg)	N/A

Abbreviations: IV, intravenous; N/A, not applicable; pt, patient; wt, weight.
Data from Bratzler DW, Dellinger EP, Olsen KM, et al. Clinical practice guidelines for antimicrobial prophylaxis in surgery. Am J Health Syst Pharm 2013;70:195–283; and Anderson DJ, Podgorny K, Berríos-Torres S, et al. Strategies to prevent surgical site infections in acute care hospitals: 2014 update. Infect Control Hosp Epidemiol 2014;35(6):605–27.

Antibiotic Prophylaxis

Timely preincisional administration of antibiotics has been found to be efficacious in the prevention of SSI (**Table 1**).[3,4,17] The recommended optimal timing for the infusion of prophylactic antibiotics is approximately 1 hour before incision, to achieve maximal tissue concentration of the agent.[3] However, newer studies have revealed that the administration of antibiotics between 0 and 30 minutes before incision is as efficacious at diminishing the rate of SSI. Agents selected should be appropriate to the procedure (eg, "clean" vs colorectal procedures) and dosage should be based on total body weight. Redosing of antimicrobial agents should occur during longer procedures or when blood loss is excessive.[3]

In conclusion, intraoperative care of the surgical patient must be conducted using a multifaceted approach. The anesthetist should be concerned not only with the psychological and physiologic welfare of the patient while undergoing an anesthetic but also with the patient's postoperative well-being. A heightened awareness is warranted regarding the role the anesthesia provider may play in the transmission of pathogens to the patient. Cognizance of the anesthetist-, patient-, and environmental-driven factors that predispose patients to the development of nosocomial infection, specifically SSI, along with knowledge of modalities to limit its occurrence, is of the utmost importance in the comprehensive care of the surgical patient. Furthermore, protection of the surgical patient against the development of HAI and SSI should encompass a collaborative effort between all members of the anesthesia and surgical teams.

REFERENCES

1. Healthcare-associated infections (HAIs). Centers for Disease Control and Prevention Web site. Available at: http://www.cdc.gov/HAI/surveillance/index.html. Accessed September 2, 2014.
2. Biddle C. Semmelweis revisited: hand hygiene and nosocomial disease transmission in the anesthesia workstation. AANA J 2009;77(3):229–37.
3. Anderson DJ, Podgorny K, Berríos-Torres S, et al. Strategies to prevent surgical site infections in acute care hospitals: 2014 update. Infect Control Hosp Epidemiol 2014;35(6):605–27.

4. Spruce L. Back to basics: preventing surgical site infections. AORN J 2014;99(5):600–8.
5. Aquino V, Holt D, Monaghan WP, et al. Examination of anesthesia equipment for the presence of blood. Poster presented at AANA Annual Congress. September 15, 2014.
6. Biddle C, Shah J. Quantification of anesthesia providers' hand hygiene in a busy metropolitan operating room: what would Semmelweis think? Am J Infect Control 2012;40:756–9.
7. Loftus RW, Koff MD, Burchman CC, et al. Transmission of pathogenic bacterial organisms in the anesthesia work area. Anesthesiology 2008;109(3):399–447.
8. Allegranzi B, Pittet D. Role of hand hygiene in healthcare-associated infection prevention. J Hosp Infect 2009;73(4):305–15.
9. Loftus RW, Muffly MK, Brown JR, et al. Hand contamination of anesthesia providers is an important risk factor for intraoperative bacterial transmission. Anesth Analg 2011;112(1):98–105.
10. Al-Hamad A, Maxwell S. How clean is clean? Proposed methods for hospital cleaning assessment. J Hosp Infect 2008;70(4):328–34. http://dx.doi.org/10.1016/j.jhin.2008.08.006.
11. Bures S, Fishbain JT, Uyehara CFT, et al. Computer keyboards and faucet handles as reservoirs of nosocomial pathogens in the intensive care unit. Am J Infect Control 2000. http://dx.doi.org/10.1067/mic.2000.107267.
12. Messina G, Quercioli C, Burgassi S, et al. How many bacteria live on the keyboard of your computer? Am J Infect Control 2011;39(7):616–7.
13. Wilson AP, Hayman S, Folan P, et al. Computer keyboards and the spread of MRSA. J Hosp Infect 2005. http://dx.doi.org/10.1016/j.jhin.2005.08.017.
14. Boyce JM, Potter-Bynow G, Chenevert C, et al. Environmental contamination due to methicillin-resistant Staphylococcus aureus: possible infection control implications. Infect Control Hosp Epidemiol 1997;18(9):622–7.
15. Anthony T, Murray BW, Sum-Ping JT, et al. Evaluating an evidence-based bundle for preventing surgical site infection: a randomized trial. Arch Surg 2011;146(3):263–9.
16. Hollmann MW, Roy RC. Antisepsis in the time of antibiotics: following in the footsteps of John Snow and Joseph Lister. Anesth Analg 2011;112(1):1–3.
17. Bratzler DW, Dellinger EP, Olsen KM, et al. Clinical practice guidelines for antimicrobial prophylaxis in surgery. Am J Health Syst Pharm 2013;70:195–283.
18. Battani J, Rosales S, Monaghan WP, et al. Personal items: a possible vector for transmission of infection as indicated by the presence of visible and occult blood. Poster presented at AANA National Convention; August 5, 2012.
19. Fukada T, Iwakiri H, Ozaki M. Anaesthetists' role in computer keyboard contamination in an operating room. J Hosp Infect 2008;70:148–53.
20. Roy RC, Brull SJ, Eichhorn JH. Surgical site infections and the anesthesia professionals' microbiome: we've all been slimed! Now what are we going to do about it? Anesth Analg 2011;112(1):4–7.
21. Melling AC, Bagar A, Scott EM, et al. Effects of preoperative warming on the incidence of wound infection after clean surgery: a randomised controlled trial. Lancet 2001. http://dx.doi.org/10.1016/S0140-6736(01)06071-8.
22. Lynch RL, Englesbe MJ, Sturm L, et al. Measurement of foot traffic in the operating room: implications for infection control. Am J Med Qual 2009;24:45–52.
23. Thiele RH, Huffmyer JL, Nemergut EC. The "six sigma" approach to the operating room environment and infection. Best Pract Res Clin Anaesthesiol 2008;22(3):537–52.

24. Weinger MB, Englund CE. Ergonomic and human factors affecting anesthetic vigilance and monitoring performance in the operating room environment. Anesthesiology 1990;73:995–1021.

25. Joga M, Palumbo EA. Removal of contaminating bacteria from computers by disinfection and hand sanitation. Am J Infect Control 2012;40:389–90.

26. Boyce JM, Pittet D. Guideline for hand hygiene in health-care settings: recommendations of the healthcare infection control practices advisory committee and the HICPAC/SHEA/APIC/IDSA hand hygiene task force. MMWR Recomm Rep 2002;51(RR-16):1–45.

27. Butterworth JF, Mackey DC, Wasnick JD. Thermoregulation, hypothermia, & malignant hyperthermia. In: Morgan and Mikhail's clinical anesthesiology. 5th edition. New York, NY: McGraw Hill Medical Education, Lange Medical Books; 2013. p. 1183–91.

Operative Care of Obstetric Patients

Marianne S. Cosgrove, CRNA, DNAP, APRN

KEYWORDS

- Obstetric anesthesia • Cesarean section • Pregnant surgical patient
- Obstetric hemorrhage

KEY POINTS

- Childbirth is the most common cause for hospitalization in the United States.
- Anesthetic care during the process of labor and delivery must account for not only the well-being of the parturient but for the fetus as well.
- The potential for complications during the process of labor and delivery range from minor to catastrophic.
- Operative care of the parturient may pose challenges to the anesthetist because of a variety of maternal and fetal factors.
- The rate of surgical delivery of the fetus, known as cesarean delivery or C-section, has increased by a factor of 60% since 1990.

INTRODUCTION

Childbirth is the most common cause for hospitalization in the United States. Approximately 4 million deliveries are performed in the United States each year. Of these, an estimated 13% experience one or more major complications during the course of labor and delivery.[1] Anesthetic care of the parturient during the process of labor and delivery may pose challenges due to several issues:

- Responsibility for the well-being of not only the mother but of the fetus
- Attention to, and allowance for, the myriad of physiologic changes that pregnancy imposes on maternal systems (**Table 1**)
- The capacity for complications ranging from minor to catastrophic during the labor process and in the immediate postpartum period

These and additional factors, such as the increasing rate of obesity in women of childbearing age, increasing maternal age, other significant comorbidities such as preexisting disease states or congenital issues, and the increasing use of assisted

Department of Anesthesiology, Yale–New Haven Hospital School of Nurse Anesthesia, Yale University, Yale Medical Group/Yale–New Haven Hospital – SRC, 1450 Chapel Street, New Haven, CT 06511, USA
E-mail address: marianne.cosgrove@yale.edu

Crit Care Nurs Clin N Am 27 (2015) 89–103
http://dx.doi.org/10.1016/j.cnc.2014.10.003
0899-5885/15/$ – see front matter © 2015 Elsevier Inc. All rights reserved.
ccnursing.theclinics.com

Table 1 Physiologic changes of pregnancy	
Cardiovascular changes	↑ HR ↑ SV ↑ CO (increases specific to trimester and stage of labor with an ~75%–80% ↑ immediately after delivery) ↓ SVR ↑ Uterine blood flow (10% of CO at term)
Respiratory changes	↑ RR; ↓ CO_2; blood pH → mild alkalosis (~7.44; kidneys waste bicarbonate to compensate for ↓ CO_2) ↑ O_2 consumption ↓ FRC (by 20% at term, greatest derangement of lung volumes and capacities) ↓ Bronchial tone ↑ VT 2° ↑ AP diameter of chest ↑ Upper airway engorgement/vascularity
Renal/endocrine/hepatic changes	↑ RBF and GFR ↓ BUN/Cr ↑ Cortisol and ACTH ↑ Aldosterone ↑ Insulin with pancreatic beta-cell hyperplasia ↓ Plasma cholinesterase ↓ Albumin (dilutional)
Neurologic changes	↑ Sedation ↓ MAC ↑ Sensitivity to local anesthetics
Gastrointestinal changes	Incompetence of gastroesophageal sphincter from ~12th week of gestation Displacement of the pylorus from the gravid uterus Delayed gastric emptying 2° pain of labor ↑ Risk of regurgitation/aspiration
Hematologic/coagulation changes	↓ H/H caused by dilutional effect of increased plasma volume ↑ 2,3 DPG (shifts oxy-Hgb dissociation curve to right; ↑ O_2 delivery) ↑ Plasma volume ↑ Synthesis of coagulation factors I, VII, VIII, IX, X, and fibrinogen ↑ Platelet size, although overall count may ↓ 2° dilution

Abbreviations: ACTH, adrenocorticotropic hormone; AP, anterior to posterior; BUN, blood urea nitrogen; CO, cardiac output; Cr, creatinine; DPG, diphosphoglycerate; FRC, functional residual capacity; GFR, glomerular filtration rate; H/H, hemoglobin and hematocrit; HR, heart rate; MAC, minimum alveolar concentration; Oxy-hgb, oxygen-hemoglobin; R, right; RBF, renal blood flow; RR, respiratory rate; SV, stroke volume; SVR, systemic vascular resistance; VT, tidal volume.

Data from Frölich MA. Maternal & fetal physiology and anesthesia. In: Butterworth JF, Mackey DC, Wasnick JD, editors. Morgan & Mikhail's Clinical Anesthesiology. New York: McGraw-Hill; 2013. p. 825–41; and Chestnut DH, Wong CA, Ysen LE, et al. Chestnut's obstetric anesthesia: principles and practice. 4th edition. Philadelphia: Elsevier Mosby; 2009.

reproductive technology (ART), must all be taken into consideration when providing anesthetic care for parturients during the potentially rigorous process of labor and delivery. This consideration may be of increased importance in parturients undergoing delivery via surgical technique.

DISCUSSION
Cesarean Section

Over the past decade, operative delivery of the fetus by way of cesarean section (C-section) has become more prevalent in the United States. According to the Centers for

Disease Control and Prevention (CDC), rates of C-section for singleton deliveries increased from 20.7% in 1996 to 32.9% in 2009, representing an overall increase of 60%.[2] However, since 2009, possibly in part due to an initiative via the American College of Obstetricians and Gynecologists (ACOG) which advocated for a more conservative approach to the delivery of infants, the rate of C-section has stabilized. Approximately 33% of deliveries in the United States were performed via C-section in 2012.[2]

There may be multiple reasons for the planned (elective) operative delivery of the fetus:

- Prior cesarean delivery
- Fetal malpresentation (breech, transverse lie)
- Multiple gestation
- Presence of placental malimplantation (previa, accreta, and variants)
- Patient request

Unplanned (semiemergent) C-section delivery of the infant may be the result of:

- Failure of the normal progression of labor
- Umbilical cord prolapse
- Maternal hemorrhage (placental abruption)
- Loss of beat-to-beat variability of fetal heart rate (FHR)/persistent nonreassuring fetal tracing
- Presence of fetal asphyxia
  - Late FHR decelerations
  - Scalp pH less than 7.2
- Prolonged rupture of amniotic membranes
- Maternal fever greater than or equal to 38°C
- Worsening status of pregnancy-induced hypertension (PIH) (seizures, development of hemolysis, elevated liver enzymes, low platelets [HELLP] syndrome)

Necessity for general endotracheal anesthesia for C-section may be the result of:

- Inability to perform regional anesthesia
  - Physical constraints (after spinal surgery, fusion, trauma)
  - Severe maternal hypotension/hemorrhage
  - Underlying or acquired coagulopathy
  - True allergy to local anesthesia (rare)
  - Patient refusal
- Catastrophic events requiring immediate delivery of the neonate (uterine rupture, amniotic fluid embolus [AFE])

When encountering actively laboring patients who request or may require anesthesia, careful preprocedural assessment and planning are crucial. This constitutes a major underpinning of the safe anesthetic care of parturients and their fetuses. Before instituting regional or general anesthesia, a comprehensive assessment of the patient via direct interview and communication with the obstetric team should include the following:

- Prior health status:
  - Past medical history (disease states, congenital defects)
  - Medications (including vitamin and herbal use)
  - Allergies
  - Past surgical history
  - Anesthetic history (personal and family)
  - Gravida and para status

- o Back pain not related to pregnancy (injury, prior surgery, presence of scoliosis, presence of hardware)
- Current health status:
  - o Age
  - o Vital signs (specifically maternal blood pressure, temperature, and fetal heart rate (FHR)/response to uterine contractions)
  - o Height, weight, body mass index (BMI) (prepregnancy and at present)
  - o Laboratory values (specifically hemoglobin, hematocrit, and platelets)
  - o Pregnancy-related issues (PIH, multiple gestations, premature fetus, placental derangements such as previa or accreta)
  - o Airway examination
  - o Progress of labor (cervical dilatation and station)
  - o Status of amniotic membranes (intact vs ruptured; time of rupture, presence of meconium)
  - o Pain score

Before the institution of either general or regional anesthesia, it is of the utmost importance to obtain a comprehensive airway assessment of the parturient. Because of the engorgement of soft tissues from increased fluid retention and vascularity, airway architecture may be distorted and tissues friable, leading to potential airway access issues.[3,4] For example, the tendency toward epistaxis may preclude the use of nasal airways to relieve acute airway obstruction. Furthermore, the increased anterior-to-posterior (AP) diameter of the maternal thoracic cage may lead to decreased access and difficulty in insertion of a laryngoscope blade into the oropharynx during laryngoscopy. This effect may be mitigated by the use of a short laryngoscope handle along with the proper positioning of the patient using the ramping technique. In addition, if a parturient who has been laboring with an epidural ultimately requires cesarean delivery, the airway should be reassessed before entering the operating suite for changes in Mallampati status.[4] As a potential consequence of receiving intravenous (IV) fluids, oxytocin, and the performance of Valsalva maneuvers repeatedly during the second (pushing) stage of labor, the tissues of the oropharynx, specifically the soft palate and tongue, may become further engorged, leading to an unanticipated difficult airway scenario. This reassessment, even in the presence of an epidural or plan for institution of spinal anesthesia before surgical delivery, remains of utmost importance in the event of regional failure.

Unanticipated difficult intubation using direct laryngoscopy in a parturient occurs with an estimated frequency of 1 in 300 patients.[5] In addition, the presence of a decreased functional residual capacity coupled with increased oxygen consumption in the parturient at term[6] may lead to a rapid rate of desaturation in the event of an inability to secure the airway in a timely manner. Because of these factors, the anesthesia provider needs to be attentive to the risks inherent in management of the airway and plan accordingly (**Table 2**).

Because of the potential for unanticipated difficult airway in parturients, regional anesthesia may be considered preferable to general endotracheal anesthesia for C-section. However, in a recent Cochrane Collaboration meta-analysis by Afolabi and Lesi[8] (2012), notwithstanding the finding that overall maternal blood loss seemed to be diminished in the regional group, there was no appreciable evidence to support the notion that regional anesthesia is superior to general anesthesia in patients with regard to major maternal or neonatal outcomes. The investigators recommended that further research to evaluate maternal outcomes, neonatal morbidity, and satisfaction with anesthetic technique is needed.[8] An 8-year retrospective review of 3430

Table 2 Preparation for airway management of the parturient	
Meticulous preprocedure airway assessment	Mallampati score Oral aperture >3 finger breadths Thyromental distance >3 finger breadths Upper lip bite test
Availability of airway equipment	Comprehensive anesthesia machine checkout Oral and intubating airways of varying sizes Face masks of varying sizes Assortment of curved and straight laryngoscope blades/short handle GlideScope Endotracheal tubes of varying sizes (small ID; flex tip) Bougies, intubating stylets Supraglottic devices (LMA Proseal, FastTrach, ILA, King) Fiberoptic bronchoscope Cricothyrotomy set
Aspiration prophylaxis	Sodium citrate 10–30 mL PO (controversial; may ↑ gastric contents/ nausea/vomiting; ↑ Na^+ load; use cautiously in PIH, renal impairment) Metoclopramide 10 mg IV slowly H_2 blocker to increase gastric pH in the event of aspiration Working suction present at HOB
Proper positioning	Parturient ramped Head of patient at level of laryngoscopist's xiphoid Left uterine displacement
Optimal preoxygenation	3–5 min of tidal volume breathing with Fio_2 1.0 or 8 vital capacity breaths more than 60 s

Abbreviations: Fio_2, fraction of inspired oxygen; HOB, head of bed; ID, internal diameter; PIH, pregnancy induced hypertension; PO, by mouth.
 Data from Refs.[5–7]

cesarean deliveries performed under general endotracheal anesthesia similarly revealed no statistically significant increase in the number of obstetric airway complications.[9] Regardless of these recent findings, parturients should always be considered at risk for regurgitation, aspiration, and unanticipated difficult or failed airway when deciding to use regional versus general anesthesia. In addition, in the case of events such as severe maternal hypotension secondary to hemorrhage or rare catastrophes such as uterine rupture or AFE, general endotracheal anesthesia is required to facilitate the expeditious delivery of the neonate.

In addition to the potential for untoward airway issues in parturients, vital signs, particularly maternal temperature, warrant the attention of the anesthesia provider. The presence of maternal fever of greater than or equal to 38°C may be the result of increased BMI, prolonged rupture of amniotic membranes, a proposed inflammatory process after the institution of epidural anesthesia,[10] or an underlying infectious process such as endometritis or chorioamnionitis.[11] This finding may suggest the need for operative delivery of the fetus because infants born to febrile mothers are at increased risk for the following issues[12]:

- Respiratory depression
- Neonatal sepsis
- Seizures
- Cerebral palsy
- Increased risk of mortality

After a comprehensive evaluation of the parturient, plans for the establishment of continuous lumbar epidural anesthesia for labor analgesia or institution of epidural, spinal, or general endotracheal anesthesia for C-section may be discussed with the patient, her significant other or family member (if appropriate and allowed by the patient), and her obstetrician and/or midwife. Acquisition of patient consent before any anesthetic procedure is of paramount importance. In the absence of an emergency scenario, time should be taken to fully explain the procedure to be used, its potential risks and benefits, and any alternative treatments that may exist. In addition, questions should be answered directly and fully and an attempt made to allay patient fears.

Care of Patients Undergoing Cesarean Section

Once it has been established that the parturient requires a cesarean delivery, care of the patient should include the following aspects[3,7,13]:

- Thorough preoperative evaluation
- Comprehensive setup:
  - Checked and fully functional anesthesia machine
  - Ancillary airway equipment
  - Working suction at the head of the bed
  - Fluids (crystalloid and colloid)
  - Fluid warmer
  - Rapid infuser
  - Blood type and screen versus crossmatch in the event of potential for hemorrhage
  - Patent IV catheter (18 gauge or better; 2 sites if potential hemorrhage is anticipated)
  - Arterial line/central venous access kits (potential hemorrhage, severe PIH, HELLP syndrome)
  - Drugs:
    - Local anesthetics (lidocaine, 2-chloroprocaine, bupivacaine, ropivacaine)
    - Pressors (ephedrine, phenylephrine, epinephrine)
    - Anticholinergics (glycopyrrolate, atropine)
    - Antihypertensives (labetalol, hydralazine)
    - Induction agents (propofol, ketamine)
    - Muscle relaxants (succinylcholine, rocuronium)
    - Antibiotics
    - Oxytocin (other uterotonics: methylergonovine and prostaglandin $F_{2\alpha}$)
    - Antiemetics (metoclopramide, ondansetron, dexamethasone)
    - Sodium citrate and H_2 blockers (famotidine)
    - Nitroglycerin (80–120 μg IV for uterine hypertonicity/retained placental fragments)
    - Intralipid 20% (treatment of local anesthetic toxicity)
  - Proper positioning of the patient
    - Left uterine displacement (LUD)
    - Ramped at head of bed
  - Ancillary O_2 via nasal cannula until delivery of the neonate (regional anesthetic)
  - End-tidal CO_2 monitor
  - Allowance for maternal support person in the operating room (OR) (regional anesthetic)

Before initiation of C-section, the patient is prepped and fully draped. If regional anesthesia is used, a T4 level is necessary to ensure adequate anesthesia for the procedure.[3,7] The process of cesarean delivery for parturients who are awake and nonsedated may constitute an extremely stressful experience. If anxiety escalates, it may precipitate events such as maternal hyperventilation that, in turn, may decrease uterine blood flow and, in extreme situations, may ultimately compromise the well-being of the fetus. The following events may contribute to increased anxiety in parturients undergoing C-section:

- Inadequate communication from the obstetrician, anesthesia provider, or OR staff
- Unfamiliar and frightening OR environment
- Discomfort:
  o Improper positioning/lack of LUD
  o Low ambient temperature in OR
  o Lack of sedation
  o Inadequate (patchy) block; breakthrough pain if uterus is exteriorized from the abdominal cavity during repair
  o Loss of sensation/feeling of dyspnea from high spinal or epidural
  o Nausea/vomiting from hypotension, unopposed parasympathetic tone from regional-induced sympathectomy
  o Intense abdominal pressure during transincisional delivery of the neonate

Taking these factors into consideration, it is evident that awake parturients are in need of constant reassurance during the operative delivery process. Furthermore, acute changes in patient status, such as failed regional or total spinal anesthesia, or catastrophic events such as uncontrolled hemorrhage, substantial venous air embolus (VAE), or AFE may indicate the need for immediate rapid sequence induction of general anesthesia using cricoid pressure and endotracheal intubation. Once the airway is secured, care must be taken to avoid hyperventilation via mechanical ventilation and maintenance of end-tidal CO_2 concentration at baseline levels.[7] These interventions preserve uterine blood flow until the fetus is delivered.

During the progress of C-section, attention must be paid to various aspects of maternal condition to assure the mother's well-being and the continued physiologic integrity of the fetus. Because placental perfusion is solely reliant on maternal blood pressure, care must be taken to maintain blood pressure via fluid administration, use of pressors if needed, and proper positioning of the parturient while undergoing C-section. Due to the presence of the gravid uterus pressing on the great vessels, supinating the parturient may lead to aortocaval compression, commonly referred to as supine hypotensive syndrome.[3,7,14] This syndrome is heralded by patient discomfort, diaphoresis, nausea and vomiting, decreased venous return, and attendant maternal tachycardia and hypotension. In extreme cases, if hypotension is sustained, maternal loss of consciousness may ensue. Fetal well-being may be compromised secondary to decreased placental perfusion; this may manifest as fetal decelerations, eventual acidosis, and neonatal depression.[14]

LUD is indicated in supine patients to alleviate the potential effects of aortocaval compression.[7,13] This position may be achieved by inserting a small wedge under the patient's right hip, thereby placing the parturient in a slight left-lateral tilted position ($\sim 15°-20°$).

Maternal hypotension may also be the result of the institution of regional anesthesia and may precipitate unpleasant symptoms such as nausea and vomiting. Prehydration with crystalloid before the inception of regional anesthesia has been advocated to attenuate potential decreases in maternal blood pressure.[3,7,13] In addition, attenuation of unopposed parasympathetic tone may be achieved with the use of glycopyrrolate 0.2 mg IV with no effect on FHR. In the past, maternal hypotension has been treated with ephedrine 5 to 10 mg IV and crystalloid bolus; however, phenylephrine 50 to 150 μg IV may safely be used with little compromise to placental blood flow as a result of uterine artery vasoconstriction.[15,16] It has been shown that neonatal cord blood pH may be higher in neonates whose mothers received phenylephrine versus repeated doses of ephedrine for the treatment of hypotension.[16] Evaluation of factors such as gravity of hypotension and maternal heart rate should also play a role in the decision as to which pressor to use.

Once the neonate has been delivered, sedation may be offered to the patient if her anxiety is untenable. The use of subhypnotic doses of propofol (10–20 mg IV), a benzodiazepine such as midazolam 1 to 2 mg IV, or nitrous oxide via face mask (40%–50%) has been advocated for anxiolysis after delivery; however, the production of amnesia during the puerperium may be undesirable to the new mother and its possibility should be discussed with the patient before instituting sedation of any kind.[13]

Plans for postoperative pain control should be made and instituted in the OR before discontinuance of the epidural catheter or emergence from general anesthesia. Use of opioids co-administered with local anesthetic in spinal or epidural anesthesia has been an efficacious and long-standing practice; however, the analgesic effects of the opioids may be short-lived and side effects such as delayed respiratory depression or pruritus may occur.[7,13] More recently, ultrasonography-guided transversus abdominis plane (TAP) blocks have been suggested for use to provide postoperative analgesia for incisional pain in patients undergoing C-section. Although initial reports reveal a reduction in postoperative opioid requirements and occurrence of nausea and vomiting,[17] administration of a TAP block requires an additional invasive procedure, and its availability may be relegated to larger teaching facilities. Sustained postoperative pain should be avoided in parturients because it may lead to an inability to bond with the newborn and participate in tasks such as breastfeeding and infant care. Interestingly, the presence of postoperative pain has recently been implicated as a contributory factor in the development of postpartum depression.[18]

Special Circumstances Surrounding Cesarean Delivery

Placenta previa

The presence of placenta previa in the parturient may require intensive preoperative preparation and planning. Previa occurs because of the partial to complete obliteration of the cervical os by an abnormally positioned placental implantation. The presence of previa may initially be discovered by ultrasonography or may be elicited by the manifestation of painless vaginal bleeding on or around the 32nd week of gestation.[7,19] The incidence of placenta previa is increasing, with an estimated occurrence of 1 in 250 pregnancies. This increase may in part be caused by the increased rate of cesarean deliveries as well as increases in maternal age and the more frequent use of ART.[20] Procedures such as in vitro fertilization are hypothesized to cause a prostaglandin-induced contraction of the uterus upon deposition of the fertilized ovum via the transcervical route. This in turn may force the embryo into the lower segment of the uterus, thereby facilitating implantation in this area.[20] Surgical delivery of the patient with placenta previa warrants prior communication between the obstetrician and the anesthetist as to surgical approach. This communication is of particular importance in cases in which the placenta is implanted on the anterior wall of the lower uterine segment, potentially requiring incision through the overlying placenta to gain access to the fetus. Preparation for these cases should include readying of blood products, establishment of dependable vascular access in the mother, and the availability of equipment such as fluid warmers and rapid infusers because blood loss may be swift and profound.[19]

Placental abruption

Placental abruption is a leading cause of maternal and perinatal morbidity and mortality. It occurs as a result of the premature separation of the placenta from the uterine wall, resulting in painful vaginal bleeding, maternal hypotension leading to shock, and fetal distress that may lead to demise. Furthermore, it is the primary causative factor in the development of disseminated intravascular coagulopathy in parturients.[21,22] In the case of retroplacental separation, the diagnosis of placental abruption may not easily be made because bleeding is not evident despite the presence of severe abdominal pain and maternal and fetal instability. Diagnosis of the presence of an occult placental abruption may be confirmed via ultrasonography. Risk factors for the development of placental abruption are as follows[7,21,22]:

- Blunt abdominal trauma (after motor vehicle accident [MVA] or fall)
- Maternal hypertension, PIH
- Multiparity
- Multiple gestation
- Advanced maternal age
- Prolonged rupture of amniotic membranes
- History of prior abruption
- Short umbilical cord
- Tobacco, alcohol, or cocaine use

Placental malimplantation

The incidence of placental malimplantations such as accreta is increasing, seeming to parallel the escalating rate of surgical deliveries.[23] Significant risk factors for the presence of placenta accreta are previous C-section and placenta previa.[22] Because the placenta does not release from the uterine wall and may fragment as a result of the accreta, the mean blood loss at delivery may be substantial and may approach 3000 to 5000 mL. If hemorrhaging from accreta or its variants (**Table 3**) is uncontrolled by conventional means such as vigorous uterine massage and uterotonic agents, treatment may ultimately require uterine artery embolization or, in extreme cases, emergency hysterectomy.[22] Although these malimplantations generally occur in known high-risk patients and may be recognized in the antepartum period via ultrasonography, occasionally accreta may be unforeseen and diagnosed at the time of delivery. This situation represents an emergent scenario and may be life threatening for obstetric patients.[22,23]

Intraoperative Complications

Although major complications in the peripartum period are rare, their onset may be abrupt and their effects and outcome severe. Despite the fact that maternal and neonatal mortalities have decreased 100-fold since the 1900s, serious obstetric complications constitute approximately 12% of all American Society of Anesthesiologists

Table 3	
Placental malimplantation subtypes	
Normal implantation	Placental implantation into stratum basalis of endometrium
Accreta	Placental implantation through stratum basalis of endometrium; minimal invasion into the myometrium
Percreta	Placental invasion into myometrium of uterus
Increta	Placental invasion through myometrium and serosa; may adhere to peritoneum and pelvic organs (bladder, bowel)

Closed Claims database claims.[7] These claims include, but are not limited to, complaints of maternal nerve injury, respiratory issues secondary to aspiration and difficult intubation, inadequate oxygenation/ventilation, newborn cerebral insult, and death. The following complications may be encountered by anesthesia providers during the intraoperative and immediate postpartum periods, and immediate recognition and treatment are crucial to the survival of both the parturient and her baby.

Venous Air Embolization

VAE is estimated to take place in more than half of all C-sections, with an occurrence rate ranging from 11% to 97%.[24] As such, C-section is considered a high-risk procedure for the development of VAE and the potential for its development must be recognized by anesthesia providers. However, most VAEs remain subclinical or may produce only minor symptoms such as transient dyspnea in the parturient. Predisposing factors for the development of VAE during delivery include uterine surgery and manipulation, hypovolemia, operative site greater than 5 cm above the heart,[24,25] and maternal positioning. Morbidity as a result of VAE is variable and depends not only on the size of the embolus but on its rate of entry into the circulation. Mortality from VAE is reported to range from 48% to 80%.[25] Although diagnosis is best made by the finding of air in the cardiac chambers via transesophageal echocardiography, the presence of VAE should be suspected in the manifestation of sudden changes in patient status during cesarean delivery. In awake patients receiving regional anesthesia, clinical presentation of entrainment of atmospheric air into the central circulation may range from complaints of mild to moderate chest discomfort and shortness of breath with hypotension to an eventual decline in oxygen saturation. Intubated patients may have profound hypotension, a sudden decrease in end-tidal CO_2 concentration, and a concomitant increase in peak inspiratory pressures caused by sudden bronchoconstriction and release of endothelial mediators of inflammation. If the presence of VAE is suspected intraoperatively, treatment should be as follows[25,26]:

- Request that the surgeon flood the field with saline
- Request that the surgeon replace the uterus into the peritoneal cavity if exteriorized for repair
- Place the patient in Trendelenburg position or left-lateral decubitus (Durant maneuver) to limit further entrainment of air into the pulmonary circulation from the right heart
- Institute positive pressure ventilation with fraction of inspired oxygen (Fio_2) 1.0 to limit entrainment of air into the pulmonary vasculature and accelerate reabsorption of nitrogen comprising the majority of the embolus
- Attempt to place a long-arm or internal/external jugular central venous catheter to aspirate air collection in right atrium
- Administer supportive measures via fluids and pressors; cardiopulmonary resuscitation if indicated

INTRAOPERATIVE AWARENESS AND RECALL

Although not life threatening, intraoperative awareness and recall is an undesirable complication that is associated with C-section under general endotracheal anesthesia. In an effort to limit fetal exposure to the effects of general anesthetics before delivery, use of lower planes of anesthesia is common for emergent C-sections. Therefore, intraoperative awareness may be an unintended consequence of this procedure.[13,27] Awareness occurs in approximately 0.4% of obstetric cases and may lead to concerns such as postpartum depression and posttraumatic stress disorder. Use of agents such as benzodiazepines that produce amnesia may be indicated after the delivery of the neonate to alleviate the incidence of awareness and recall.[13]

POSTPARTUM BLEEDING AND HEMORRHAGE AFTER CESAREAN SECTION

There are many factors that contribute to the presence of postpartum bleeding and hemorrhage after surgical delivery. The typical estimated blood loss after peripartum procedures is listed in **Table 4**.

Causes of peripartum hemorrhage may be easily recalled by using the "4 Ts" mnemonic:

- Tone (atonia of the uterus)
- Tissue (retained placenta, placental malimplantation)
- Trauma (cervical or vaginal lacerations, placental abruption, uterine inversion or rupture)
- Thrombin (underlying or acquired coagulopathies)

Atonia of the uterus is the most frequent cause of postpartum hemorrhage, occurring in approximately 2% to 5% of all deliveries.[28] Factors contributing to the development of uterine atony and subsequent bleeding include:

- Uterine overdistention from multiple gestation or polyhydramnios
- Use of oxytocin to induce labor
- Retained placental fragments
- Maternal diabetes with fetal macrosomia
- Multiparity
- Extended use of tocolytic agents
- Use of volatile agents

Uterine atony may initially be treated by fundal massage and administration of uterotonic agents (**Table 5**). Of the pharmacologic agents used to treat uterine atony, oxytocin (Pitocin) is regarded as a first-line agent. Oxytocin, an endogenous hormone secreted by the posterior pituitary, regulates uterine contractility during the labor process and after delivery. A bolus dose of 3 to 10 U IV of oxytocin immediately after placental delivery via cesarean has been advocated to decrease overall postpartum bleeding and provide prophylaxis against postpartum hemorrhage. However, studies regarding the efficacy and safety of this maneuver are contradictory. Although Davies and colleagues[29] (2005) found no hemodynamic change associated with the rapid bolus of 10 U of oxytocin at delivery, other studies have revealed the occurrence of side effects such as ST-T depression, tachycardia, hypotension, chest pain, and myocardial ischemia.[30,31] Despite the efficacy of this maneuver in increasing uterine tone expeditiously, the potential for serious side effects from its use facilitates a

Table 4 Mean blood loss after delivery	
Delivery	**Blood Loss (mL)**
Vaginal (singleton)	500
Uncomplicated cesarean birth	1000
Cesarean hysterectomy	1500

Data from Gabbe SG, Niebyl JR, Simpson JL, et al. Obstetrics: normal and problem pregnancies. 6th edition. Philadelphia: Saunders; 2012.

Table 5
Uterotonic agents

Uterotonic Agent	Dose	Potential Untoward Effects
Hormone: Oxytocin (Pitocin)	IV infusion of 20–80 U/L crystalloid Prebolus 3–10 U IV (controversial)	Nausea/vomiting, flushing, hypotension, tachycardia, chest pain, ST segment changes with rapid administration
Ergot alkaloid: Methylergonovine (Methergine)	0.2 mg IM or slow IV (IM preferred)	Hypertension; contraindicated for use in PIH Tachycardia Seizures
Prostaglandin: 15-Methylprostaglandin F$_{2\alpha}$ (Hemabate/carboprost tromethamine)	250 μg IM or intramyometrial	Bronchoconstriction; contraindicated for use in asthmatics Allergic reaction Headache

Abbreviation: IM, intramuscular.
Data from Refs.[28–31]

high risk/benefit ratio that may not support its use routinely. In the case of potential for postpartum hemorrhage, such as with multiple gestations or placental issues, the use of a preinfusion bolus of oxytocin 3 to 10 U IV may be applicable.

If oxytocin proves to be ineffective in the treatment of uterine hypotonicity, other medications such as methylergonovine, an ergot alkaloid, or prostaglandin derivatives such as carboprost tromethamine, may be administered. Although potentially more potent in producing uterine tone, these agents may have untoward side effects and must be used with caution in certain patient populations (see **Table 5**).

Anesthetic Care of the Obstetric Patient for Nonobstetric Surgery

On occasion, pregnant patients present for surgery for nonobstetric procedures. In the United States, there are approximately 75,000 surgeries per year performed on pregnant patients.[32] Although procedures such as liver transplantation, craniotomy, and cardiopulmonary bypass have been successfully performed on these patients with good fetal outcomes,[33] the following procedures represent the most frequently performed operations in pregnant patients:

- Cholecystectomy
- Ovarian cystectomy
- Appendectomy
- Breast procedures
- Cervical cerclage (for history of spontaneous abortion)

Factors such as the physiologic changes of pregnancy coupled with fetal well-being are of paramount importance when caring for pregnant surgical patients. Specific attention should be paid to the following factors when planning the anesthetic course for these patients[32,33]:

- Thorough preoperative evaluation:
  - Patient history
    - Week of gestation
    - Airway examination
  - Fetal condition (FHR)

- Communication with surgeon as to procedural plan and requirements
- Postponement of surgery until the second trimester of pregnancy if nonemergent
- Use of regional anesthesia if possible to limit fetal exposure to anesthetic agents
- Avoidance of potentially teratogenic agents, particularly during the period of organogenesis ($\sim$ 15–58 days)
- Use of aspiration precautions
- Proper positioning of patient with LUD instituted by 18th to 20th week of gestation
- Maintenance of normocarbia if the patient is intubated/ventilated
- Maintenance of maternal blood pressure and avoidance of hypoxemia

Although past recommendations have advocated the avoidance of agents such as benzodiazepines and nitrous oxide in pregnant surgical patients, newer references suggest that most drugs used during the course of anesthesia are potentially safe if used judiciously. To date, acute exposure to anesthetic agents has not been shown to precipitate fetal abnormalities.[32,33] However, despite the relaxing effects of the volatile anesthetics on the uterus, the incidence of premature labor on recovery is increased at approximately 8% to 11%. This occurrence increases in conjunction with pelvic procedures and it constitutes the major complication associated with surgery in pregnant patients.[32]

While caring for pregnant surgical patients, careful attention to maternal positioning with LUD, maintenance of blood pressure, normal end-tidal CO_2 concentration, and ample oxygenation are crucial as these interventions serve to maintain placental blood flow and avoid the potential for the development of fetal asphyxia. Parenteral medications such as opioids may be given safely, and postoperative pain control is of the utmost importance. Because of the nature of fetal circulation, the fetus experiences limited exposure to parenteral medications. Therefore, the benefit of the analgesic effect of postoperative opioids may offset the untoward symptoms of acute pain in pregnant patients, such as stress, hyperventilation, and hypertension, all of which may compromise fetal well-being.[33]

SUMMARY

The operative care of pregnant patients, whether for delivery of the neonate or for nonobstetric surgical procedures, must take into consideration many variables. An awareness of maternal physiologic changes, fetal requirements, effects of anesthetic agents on both the mother and the fetus, and the potential for complications ranging from mild to life threatening is essential for obstetric anesthetists. In addition, a comprehensive evaluation of the parturient, ample preparation of drugs and equipment in the operative suite, and cooperation with the obstetrician and the surgical team are of major importance in ensuring the safe and effective anesthetic care of this special patient population.

REFERENCES

1. Glance LG, Dick AW, Glantz C, et al. Rates of major obstetrical complications vary almost fivefold among US hospitals. Health Aff 2014;33(8):1330–6.
2. Osterman MJ, Martin JA. Changes in cesarean delivery rates by gestational age: United States, 1996–2011. NCHS Data Brief 2013;124:1–8.
3. Chestnut DH, Wong CA, Ysen LE, et al. Chestnut's obstetric anesthesia: principles and practice. 4th edition. Philadelphia: Elsevier Mosby; 2009.

4. Kodali BS, Chandrasekhar S, Bulich LN, et al. Airway changes during labor and delivery. Anesthesiology 2008;108:357–62.
5. Mhyre JM, Healy D. The unanticipated difficult intubation in obstetrics. Anesth Analg 2011;112(3):648–52.
6. Frölich MA. Maternal & fetal physiology and anesthesia. In: Butterworth JF, Mackey DC, Wasnick JD, editors. Morgan & Mikhail's clinical anesthesiology. New York: McGraw-Hill; 2013. p. 825–41.
7. Frölich MA. Obstetric anesthesia. In: Butterworth JF, Mackey DC, Wasnick JD, editors. Morgan & Mikhail's clinical anesthesiology. New York: McGraw-Hill; 2013. p. 825–41.
8. Afolabi BB, Lesi FE. Regional versus general anaesthesia for Caesarean section. Cochrane Database Syst Rev 2012;(10):CD004350. http://dx.doi.org/10.1002/14651858.CD004350.pub3.
9. Djabatey EA, Barclay PM. Difficult and failed intubation in 3430 obstetric general anaesthetics. Anaesthesia 2009;64:1168.
10. Goetzl L. Epidural fever in obstetric patients: it's a hot topic [editorial]. Anesth Analg 2014;118(3):494–5.
11. Chen KT. Intrapartum fever. UpToDate. Available at: http://www.uptodate.com/contents/intrapartum-fever. Accessed July 31, 2014.
12. American Heart Association (AHA). Neonatal resuscitation guidelines. Circulation 2005;112:IV188–95. http://dx.doi.org/10.1161/CIRCULATIONAHA.105.166574.
13. Grant GJ. Anesthesia for Cesarean delivery. UpToDate. Available at: http://www.uptodate.com/contents/anesthesia-for-cesarean-delivery#H13721019. Accessed July 5, 2014.
14. Kinsella SM, Lohmann G. Supine hypotensive syndrome. Obstet Gynecol 1994;83(5):774–88.
15. Lee A, Ngan Kee WD, Gin T. A quantitative, systematic review of randomized controlled trials of ephedrine versus phenylephrine for the management of hypotension during spinal anesthesia for cesarean delivery. Anesth Analg 2002;94:920.
16. Ngan Kee WD, Khaw KS, Lau TK, et al. Randomised double-blind comparison of phenylephrine vs. ephedrine for maintaining blood pressure during spinal anesthesia for non-elective Caesarean section. Anaesthesia 2008;63:1319.
17. Baaj JM, Alsatli RA, Majaj HA, et al. Efficacy of ultrasound-guided transversus abdominis plane (TAP) block for postcesarean section delivery analgesia–a double-blind, placebo-controlled, randomized study. Middle East J Anesthesiol 2010;20(6):821–6.
18. Wisner CL, Stika CS, Clark CT. Double duty: does epidural labor analgesia reduce both pain and postpartum depression? [editorial]. Anesth Analg 2014;119(2):219–21.
19. Woods SN, Shabaz PW, Lindeman KS. Placenta previa. In: Fleisher LA, Roizen MF, editors. The essence of anesthesia practice. 3rd edition. Philadelphia: Saunders; 2010. p. 294.
20. Romundstad LB, Bente L, Romundstad PR, et al. Increased risk of placenta previa in pregnancies following IVF/ICSI; a comparison of ART and non-ART pregnancies in the same mother. Humanit Rep 2006;21(9):2353–8.
21. Gibbs CP. Abruptio placentae. In: Fleisher LA, Roizen MF, editors. The essence of anesthesia practice. 3rd edition. Philadelphia: Saunders; 2010. p. 2.
22. Gabbe SG, Niebyl JR, Simpson JL, et al. Obstetrics: normal and problem pregnancies. 6th edition. Philadelphia: Saunders; 2012.

23. The American College of Obstetrics and Gynecology (ACOG). Committee opinion: placenta accreta. 2012. Available at: http://www.acog.org/Resources-And-Publications/Committee-Opinions/Committee-on-Obstetric-Practice/Placenta-Accreta. Accessed August 2, 2014.
24. Lowenwirt IP, Chi DS, Handwerker SM. Nonfatal venous air embolism during cesarean section: a case report and review of the literature. Obstet Gynecol Surv 1994;49(1):72.
25. Shaikh N, Ummunisa F. Acute management of vascular air embolism. J Emerg Trauma Shock 2009;2(3):180–5. http://dx.doi.org/10.4103/0974-2700.55330.
26. Gordy S, Rowell S. Vascular air embolism. Int J Crit Illn Inj Sci 2013;3(1):73–6.
27. Duke J. Awareness during anesthesia. In: Anesthesia secrets, 4th edition. Philadelphia, PA: Mosby Elsevier; vol. 29. 2011; p. 207-9.
28. Donnelly J. Maternal hemorrhage: etiology and management. Curr Rev Nurs Anesth 2012;34(21):253–64.
29. Davies JA, Tessier JL, Woodman MC, et al. Maternal hemodynamics after oxytocin bolus compared with infusion in the third stage of labor: a randomized controlled trial. Obstet Gynecol 2005;105(2):294–9.
30. Jonsson M, Hanson U, Lidell C, et al. ST depression at caesarean section and the relation to oxytocin dose. A randomized controlled trial. BJOG 2010;117:76.
31. Bhattacharya S, Ghosh S, Ray D, et al. Oxytocin administration during cesarean delivery: randomized controlled trial to compare intravenous bolus with intravenous infusion regimen. J Anaesthesiol Clin Pharmacol 2013;29:32–5.
32. Kamel I. The pregnant surgical patient. In: Fleisher LA, Roizen MF, editors. The essence of anesthesia practice. Philadelphia: Saunders; 2011.
33. Norwitz ER, Park JS, Snegovskikh D. Management of the pregnant patient undergoing nonobstetric surgery. UpToDate. Available at: http://www.uptodate.com/contents/management-of-the-pregnant-patient-undergoing-nonobstetric-surgery. Accessed August 18, 2014.

Pediatric Emergencies

Erin Ryan, CRNA, MS, APRN

KEYWORDS

• Pediatric • Emergencies • Medications • Pathophysiology • Management

KEY POINTS

- The Pediatric Assessment Triangle is a useful tool for the critical care nurse to assess a child in an emergency situation.
- Pediatric patients require accurate and effective medication dosing, based on height and/ or weight.
- Pediatric emergencies are unique and require the critical care nurse to possess necessary information to provide the highest level of care.

INTRODUCTION

Pediatric patients are not simply small adults. They present with unique anatomy, physiology, and pathophysiology. Taking this into consideration, it is imperative for the critical care nurse to have a thorough understanding of the pediatric patient's needs and be able to provide specialized care, especially during emergency situations. This article reviews the assessment of the pediatric patient, accurate medication dosing of the pediatric patient examining both height and weight as measures, and Pediatric Advanced Life Support (PALS). Specific pediatric emergencies are reviewed according to organ systems, with a focus on definition, presentation, pathophysiology, management, and special considerations. The examples of pediatric emergencies are applicable to a variety of age ranges.

Assessment of the Pediatric Patient

Assessment of the pediatric patient with an acute illness or injury requires special knowledge and skills. Scoring methodologies and severity scales can lack precision in the pediatric patient. A model tool for assessment of all children is the Pediatric Assessment Triangle (PAT). It is a simple, reproducible, and useful tool for children of all ages with all levels of illness and injury severity. The PAT assists the critical care nurse with early recognition and prioritization of problems as a basis for organized resuscitation, support, and treatment.[1]

The PAT (**Fig. 1**)[2] is a simple tool designed for the initial assessment of any pediatric patient. Using visual clues, the nurse is able to assess the severity of the

The author has no disclosures.
Department of Anesthesiology, Yale-New Haven Hospital, 20 York Street, New Haven, CT 06510, USA
E-mail address: erinr309@comcast.net

Crit Care Nurs Clin N Am 27 (2015) 105–120
http://dx.doi.org/10.1016/j.cnc.2014.10.007 ccnursing.theclinics.com
0899-5885/15/$ – see front matter © 2015 Elsevier Inc. All rights reserved.

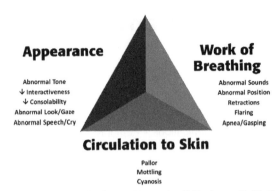

Fig. 1. Pediatric assessment triangle. (*From* Horeczko T, Enriquez B, McGrath NE, et al. The pediatric assessment triangle: accuracy of its application by nurses in the triage of children. J Emerg Nurs 2013;39(2):182–9. http://dx.doi.org/10.1016/j.jen.2011; with permission.)

patient's illness or injury and urgency for treatment. The 3 components of the PAT are overlapping, interdependent, and reflective of the pediatric patient's physiologic status.[1]

The PAT uses 3 key features of pediatric cardiopulmonary assessment: (1) appearance, (2) work of breathing, and (3) circulation to skin. Appearance is the single most important parameter when assessing the severity of illness or injury. Appearance is a reflection of the adequacy of ventilation, oxygenation, brain perfusion, homeostasis, and central nervous system function. Components of appearance include *tone*, *interactability*, *consolability*, *look/gaze*, and *speech/cry* (TICLS). Although appearance reflects the presence of illness or injury, it does not indicate the source of distress, unlike work of breathing and circulation to skin. These elements provide specific information about physiologic instability. Work of breathing is a reflection of the pediatric patient's compensation to cardiopulmonary stress. The critical care nurse assesses work of breathing by listening for abnormal airway sounds and observing breathing effort, position, retraction, flaring, and apnea/gasping. A circulatory assessment determines the adequacy of cardiac output and perfusion of vital organs. Pallor, mottling, and cyanosis are key visual indicators of reduced circulation to skin and the overall status of circulation to the body's end organs.[1] By successfully combining the different characteristics of the PAT, the critical care nurse can rapidly establish a degree of severity and identify the likely physiologic abnormality and begin resuscitation.[1]

Box 1
Estimating the pediatric patient's weight

Average birth weight = 3.5 kg

Infants (5 months) = birth weight × 2 = 7 kg

Infants (1 year) = birth weight × 3 = 10.5 kg

Greater than 1 year = 8 + (age in years × 2) = weight (kilograms)

If the patient's weight is known in pounds, divide by 2.2 for kilograms.

Adapted from Dieckmann R, Brownstein D, Gausche-Hill M. The pediatric assessment triangle: a novel approach for the rapid evaluation of children. Pediatr Emerg Care 2010;26(4):312–5.

Resuscitation of the Pediatric Patient

Managing pediatric resuscitation requires precision and a systematic approach.[3] Dosages of pediatric medications are typically weight based. In an emergency situation, the critical care nurse may not have an accurate patient weight. There are multiple means for calculating dosages in the pediatric patient, including estimating the patient's weight (**Box 1**) and using a length-based tape (**Box 2**). Regardless of the method used a thorough understanding of appropriate drug dosages for the pediatric patient is necessary in an emergency situation.

The correlation between length and weight is well established and applied to both the 50th percentile curves and the Broselow Pediatric Emergency Tape. The tape uses length-based calculation to estimate patient weight, allowing health care providers to meet the resuscitation and medication needs of the pediatric patient. Specifically, the tape is designed for children younger than 12 years, with weight up to 36 kg, and height between 46 and 143 cm. The tape uses color-coded zones that allow providers, such as critical care nurses, to quickly determine a baseline of resuscitation equipment and medication.[3]

Despite recent concerns regarding inaccuracies when using a length-based tool with today's overweight population, the Broselow tape is a useful tool for the pediatric patient. Research has demonstrated that the Broselow tape is the most reliable predictor in most situations. Furthermore, the American Heart Association (AHA) is clear that resuscitation medications used for PALS should be based on the pediatric patient's weight, and if it is unknown, then it is reasonable to use a length tape with precalculated doses.[3] The AHA confirms that cardiac arrest in infants and children does not usually result from a primary cardiac condition. More often, it is the terminal result of progressive respiratory failure or shock, also called asphyxial arrest. Asphyxia begins with a variable period of systemic hypoxemia, hypercapnea, and acidosis, progresses to bradycardia and hypotension, and culminates with cardiac arrest. It is imperative that the critical care nurse aggressively implements the evidence-based resuscitation guidelines, as they may improve outcomes significantly during in-hospital cardiac arrests, such as in the operating room. Appendices 1–3 depict the AHA's algorithms for cardiac arrest, bradycardia, and tachycardia in the pediatric patient, respectively.[4]

Pediatric Emergencies

Pediatric patients of various ages and sizes present with various illnesses, injuries, and emergencies. The most common pediatric emergencies, which the critical care nurse may be faced with in the operating room setting, are the focus of the next section. The information aides the critical care nurse caring for the emergent pediatric patient to be able to recognize the acutely ill or injured child, initiate appropriate treatment, and maintain and enhance skills.[5]

Neurologic Emergencies

Primary neurologic injury in pediatric patients can be induced by diverse intrinsic and extrinsic factors including brain trauma, tumors, and intracranial infections. Increased intracranial pressure (ICP) as a result of the primary injury or delayed treatment may lead to secondary (preventable) brain injury. Present management strategies to improve survival and neurologic outcome focus on reducing ICP while optimizing cerebral perfusion and meeting cerebral metabolic demands.[6]

ICP is determined by the total force exerted by the brain, blood, and cerebrospinal fluid contained within the fixed volume of the skull. Normal values for ICP increase with

Box 2
Broselow pediatric emergency tape

Gray
Age: 0 to 2 months
Weight: 3 to 5 kg
Length: less than 59.5 cm

Pink
Age: 3 to 6 months
Weight: 6 to 7 kg
Length: 59.5 to 66.5 cm

Red
Age: 7 to 10 months
Weight: 8 to 9 kg
Length: 66.5 to 74 cm

Purple
Age: 11 to 18 months
Weight: 10 to 11 kg
Length: 74 to 84.5 cm

Yellow
Age: 18 to 36 months
Weight: 12 to 14 kg
Length: 84.5 to 97.5 cm

White
Age: 3 to 4 years
Weight: 15 to 18 kg
Length: 97.5 to 110 cm

Blue
Age: 5 to 6 years
Weight: 19 to 22 kg
Length: 110 to 122 cm

Orange
Age: 7 to 9 years
Weight: 24 to 28 kg
Length: 122 to 137 cm

Green
Age: 10 to 12 years
Weight: 30 to 36 kg
Length: 137 to 150 cm

Data from Moses S. Broselow tape. Family practice notebook. 2012. Available at: http://www.drbits.net/ER/Pharm/BrslwTp.htm. Accessed August 31, 2014.

$$Cerebral\ Perfusion\ Pressure = Mean\ Arterial\ Pressure - Intracranial\ Pressure$$

Fig. 2. Cerebral perfusion pressure formula. (*Data from* Pitfield AF, Carroll AB, Kissoon N. Emergency management of increased intracranial pressure. Pediatr Emerg Care 2012;28(2):200–4.)

age, from 6 mm Hg in infants to 10 to 15 mm Hg in adults. Compensatory mechanisms exist, but once the limits are exceeded, ICP increases. Increased ICP may cause cerebral ischemia by decreasing cerebral perfusion pressure and thereby cerebral blood flow to critical levels (**Fig. 2**).[6]

The pediatric patient with a neurologic emergency (elevated ICP) can present with various historical features, symptoms, and signs (**Table 1**) that the critical care nurse recognizes as neurologic compromise.[6]

The critical care nurse uses the PAT to assess airway, breathing, and circulation for the pediatric patient with potential neurologic insults. Airway protection must be ensured for patients with an altered level of consciousness, as well as normal oxygenation and ventilation, and normocarbia. Furthermore, the pediatric patient's blood pressure should be maintained with aggressive fluid resuscitation using crystalloids. Additional management of the pediatric patient with neurologic insult includes seizure control, such as the administration of anticonvulsants and protective positioning; sedation; analgesia; hyperventilation; and hyperosmolar therapies. Postoperatively, it is important to maintain normoglycemia and normonatremia and to maintain the head midline and elevated at 30°, which lowers ICP without lowering cerebral perfusion pressure. Furthermore, cooling blankets and other means to lower cerebral metabolic demand can be used to lower body temperature. It is also important to monitor and maintain cerebrospinal fluid drainage systems, such as ventriculostomies or lumbar drains.[6]

Ear, Nose, and Throat Emergencies

Children are constantly exploring their surroundings and are apt to present to the operating room with various ear, nose, and throat (ENT) emergencies, such as foreign bodies, trauma, abscesses, mastoiditis, posttonsillectomy complications, and epistaxis. Unrecognized ENT emergencies in the pediatric patient can result in aspiration, complete airway obstruction, hemorrhage, and permanent tissue injury. Present management strategies prioritize maintaining a patent airway, effective ventilation, and preserving hemodynamic stability. **Table 2** summarizes common pediatric ENT emergencies.[7]

Table 1		
Historical features, symptoms, and signs of increased ICP		
Historical Features	**Symptoms**	**Signs**
History of trauma	Headache	Ataxia
Previous VP shunt	Diplopia	Seizures
Bleeding diathesis	Nausea	Pupillary asymmetry
Morning vomiting		Decreased LOC
Nocturnal headache		
Developmental regression		

Abbreviations: LOC, level of consciousness; VP, ventriculoperitoneal.
Adapted from Pitfield AF, Carroll AB, Kissoon N. Emergency management of increased intracranial pressure. Pediatr Emerg Care 2012;28(2):200–4.

Table 2
Pediatric ENT emergencies

Emergency	Presentation	Pathophysiology	Management	Considerations
Foreign bodies	Foreign body in nasal passages, ear canals, mouth Increased work of breathing, stridor, or respiratory failure	Epistaxis Unilateral drainage Aspiration Airway compromise	Irrigation Removal Positive pressure Magill forceps	Need for sedation Trauma Bleeding Destruction/granulation from chronic foreign body Airway maintenance
Trauma	Oral/posterior pharynx injuries Nasal injuries Decrease oral intake Drooling, Bloody emesis	Blunt trauma Proximity to internal carotid artery Airway compromise	Keep patient calm Emergency airway equipment available Airway maintenance	Need for sedation Bleeding
Abscesses	Fever Neck pain Sore throat Difficulty swallowing Decreased oral intake Drooling Muffled voice	Collection of fluid, Erythema Asymmetric swelling Bulging soft tissue Airway deviation Sepsis Hemorrhage Lemierre syndrome	Surgical drainage, Hydration Pain control Antibiotics Airway maintenance	Airway obstruction Progression of illness Aspiration pneumonia Thrombosis Aneurysm

Mastoiditis	Acute otitis media complication with downward and outward protrusion of auricle and erythema over mastoid process	Temporal bone sinuses Hearing loss Labrynthitis/dizziness Cranial nerve VII involvement with facial nerve paralysis Meningitis Cerebral thrombosis	Broad-spectrum antibiotics Anticoagulation therapy	Vague symptoms: Headache Papilledema Vomiting Cranial nerve VI paralysis
Posttonsillectomy complications	Hemorrhaging Primary: within the first 24 h Secondary: 1 wk postprocedure	Inadequate hemostasis Eschar removal Dehydration	Control bleeding Fluid resuscitation Blood resuscitation Pain control	Respiratory depression with swollen posterior pharynx Upper airway obstruction Death
Epistaxis	Nasal bleeding Digital or blunt trauma Mucosal irritation from URI	Anterior: Most common Kisselbach plexus Posterior: Most profuse bleeding Sphenopalatine artery Airway compromise Hemodynamic instability Aspiration	Suctioning Vasoconstrictors Applied pressure with head forward from 5–15 min Balloon/tamponade for posterior bleeds Airway maintenance	Bleeding

Abbreviation: URI, upper respiratory tract infection.
Adapted from Stoner MJ, Dulaurier M. Pediatric ENT emergencies. Emerg Med Clin North Am 2013;31(3):795–808.

The PAT can be used to assess airway, breathing, and circulation for the pediatric patient with potential ENT complications. The immediate priority is maintaining a patent airway and effective ventilation. The critical care nurse also ensures that the pediatric ENT patient has intravenous access, appropriate laboratory blood drawn, and blood products available. Emergency airway equipment availability is necessary should the patient require an advanced or surgical airway.

Cardiac Emergencies

Cardiac disease is uncommon in pediatric patients but is divided into structural disease, conduction abnormalities, and acquired illnesses. Structural congenital heart disease are further divided into cyanotic and acyanotic categories, conduction abnormalities are classified as new-onset illness or postprocedure, and acquired illnesses may include myocarditis, endocarditis, pericarditis, Kawasaki disease, and cardiomyopathies. Timely identification, management, and stabilization of these patients are important goals for the critical care nurse.[8] **Table 3** summarizes pediatric cardiac emergencies.

A thorough assessment of pediatric cardiac patients, listening to heart sounds, and examining both electrocardiogram and chest radiographs are warranted for this patient population. The immediate priority is stabilizing the patient and preventing further decompensation. The critical care nurse also confirms that the pediatric cardiac patient has intravenous access, including central lines for caustic inotropes or vasopressors, as well as hemodynamic monitoring, appropriate laboratory blood drawn, and blood products available.

Respiratory Emergencies

Acute respiratory distress is one of the most common crises encountered by pediatric critical care nurses. Severity can range from mild, self-limiting illness to life-threatening disease.[9] Infants with respiratory illness are at a greater risk from their higher oxygen consumption, smaller functional residual capacity, and greater airway resistance. Softer cartilaginous airway components and muscle fatigue also contribute to pediatric patients developing respiratory failure. The most common respiratory emergencies are presented in **Table 4**.

The critical care nurse can use the PAT to assess airway, breathing, and circulation for the pediatric patient with potential respiratory emergencies, which allows the provider to quickly identify evidence of increased respiratory effort, including tachypnea; accessory muscle use; intercostal, subcostal, or suprasternal retractions; and abnormal sounds such as stridor, wheeze, or grunting. Further evidence of respiratory distress may include difficulty talking or feeding, diminished breath sounds, agitation, confusion, or decreased level of consciousness.[5] The immediate priority is maintaining a patent airway and effective ventilation. It is important to have emergency airway equipment available should the patient require an advanced or surgical airway.

Other Pediatric Emergencies

It is important to consider the variety of emergencies that occur in an operating room. Other emergencies may include, but are not limited to, sepsis, trauma, burns, and neonatal emergencies. Each is a unique situation during which the critical care nurse must thoroughly assess the patient and possess a thorough understanding of the pathophysiology to provide the highest level of care. These emergencies are presented in **Table 5**.

Table 3
Pediatric cardiac emergencies

Emergency	Presentation	Pathophysiology	Management	Considerations
Cyanotic heart disease	Cyanosis ± Respiratory distress Murmur Feeding difficulties CHF Pulmonary disease	Tetralogy of Fallot Transposition of the great arteries Total anomalous pulmonary venous return Tricuspid atresia Truncus arteriosus	Oxygen therapy Gentle fluid resuscitation PGE_1 Palliative surgical repair Acid-base balance	Apnea Hypotension Need for sedation Mechanical ventilation Vasopressors Inotropes
Acyanotic heart disease	CHF Chamber enlargement Feeding difficulties Poor weight gain Pulmonary hypertension Murmur Valvular regurgitation	Left-to-right shunt lesions: Ventricular septal defects Atrial septal defects Patent ductus arteriosus Endocardial cushion defects	Surgical intervention	
Aortic structural defects	Shock Metabolic acidosis Decreased lower extremity pulses CHF Murmur	Coarctation of the aorta Hypoplastic left heart syndrome Aortic stenosis	PGE_1 Stabilization of patient Surgical correction	Intubation Mechanical ventilation Diuretics Inotropes
Acquired disease	Vomiting Decreased activity Poor feeding CHF Tachycardia Tachypnea Gallop rhythm Decreased heart sounds Chest pain Fever Erythema	Myocarditis: Infectious Autoimmune Toxin-mediated Pericarditis: Viral Bacterial Endocarditis: Bacterial Kawasaki disease Cardiomyopathy	Identify cause Treat cause Treat CHF Control arrhythmias	Oxygen therapy Diuretics Inotropes ACE inhibitors Immunoglobulin Antibiotics Pain management

For information regarding arrhythmias, refer to Appendices 1–3.
Abbreviations: ACE, acetylcholinesterase; CHF, congestive heart failure; PGE_1, prostaglandin E1.
Adapted from Barata IA. Cardiac emergencies. Emerg Med Clin North Am 2013;31(3):677–704.

Table 4
Pediatric respiratory emergencies

Emergency	Presentation	Pathophysiology	Management	Considerations
Asthma[5,9]	Wheezing Coughing Chest tightness Bronchospasm, Shortness of breath	Chronic disease of lower airways Hyperresponsiveness to stimuli leading to bronchial smooth muscle constriction Inflammation Edema IgE-mediated: allergen-triggered Non-IgE-mediated: NSAIDs Exercise Cold-triggered	Monitor oxygen saturation Oxygen therapy Short-acting beta agonist: Nebulizer Metered-dose inhaler (albuterol) Muscarinic acetylcholine receptor blocker: Atrovent Corticosteroids	Intravenous access Fluid resuscitation Anesthetics: Ketamine Sevoflurane
Foreign body aspiration[5]	Varies with: Size Position Mobility of foreign body Time of inhalation Cough Wheeze Dyspnea, Stridor Voice change Fever Productive cough Respiratory distress	Foreign body Air-trapping Hyperinflation of affected side	Assessing severity/patient's ability to cough Back blows CPR/PALS Bag-mask ventilation Definitive treatment: Removal via rigid bronchoscopy	Emergency airway equipment Ventilating bronchoscope

Condition	Signs/Symptoms	Cause/Complications	Treatment	Comments
Laryngospasm[10]	Partial: Inspiratory stridor; Complete: Absent breath sounds, Tracheal tug, Paradoxic movement: Chest, Abdomen; Late signs: Desaturation, Bradycardia, Cyanosis	Stimulation of afferent fibers of superior laryngeal nerve resulting in reflex closure of upper airway due to glottis musculature spasm; Hypoxia, Hypercapnea, Arrhythmia, Cardiac arrest, Pulmonary edema, Bronchospasm, Gastric aspiration	Jaw thrust, Oral or nasal airway, Positive pressure ventilation with 100% oxygen, Deepen anesthetic: IV or inhalational, Succinylcholine 0.1–3 mg IV ±, Atropine 0.02 mg/kg IV	Avoidance of patient stimulation during stage 2 of anesthesia
Medical emergencies[5,9]	Fever, Cough, Hoarseness, Stridor, Tachypnea, Increased respiratory effort, Wheezing, Lethargy, Irritability	Croup, Bronchiolitis, Pneumonia, Epiglottitis, Other infectious process	Oxygen therapy, Intubation, Corticosteroids, Nebulized epinephrine, Fluid resuscitation, Antibiotics	Ill patients are not usually brought to the operating room but may be present in an emergency

Abbreviations: CPR, cardiopulmonary resuscitation; IV, intravenous; NSAID, nonsteroidal anti-inflammatory drug.
Data from Refs.[5,9,10].

Table 5
Other pediatric emergencies

Emergency	Presentation	Pathophysiology	Management	Considerations
Sepsis	Hypothermia Hyperthermia Inadequate tissue perfusion Altered mental status Prolonged capillary refill Diminished pulses Cool peripheries Bounding peripheral pulses Wide pulse pressure Decreased urine output	Bacterial infection: meningococcal	Resuscitation Maintenance or restoration of airway, oxygenation, ventilation, and circulation Boluses of 20 mL/kg of isotonic fluid	Inotropes Intubation Mechanical ventilation Central venous access
Trauma	Peripheral circulatory restriction Tachycardia (without hypotension) Confusion Prolonged capillary refill	Hypovolemia secondary to blunt trauma Hemorrhage secondary to penetrating trauma Airway compromise	Airway management Stabilization of cervical spine Peripheral vascular/intraosseous access Boluses of 20 mL/kg of isotonic fluid Blood after 40 mL/kg of crystalloid	Considered full stomach Risk of nausea and vomiting Bradycardia may indicate head injury Pain management
Burns	First, second or third degree burns Peripheral vasoconstriction Prolonged capillary refill	Systemic inflammatory response Decreased pulmonary function Profound hypovolemia	Airway management Ventilation Vascular/intraosseous access Fluid management: Modified Parkland formula Analgesia	Smoke inhalation Carbon monoxide poisoning Upper airway obstruction: Inhalational injury Immediate or early intubation
Neonatal emergencies	Feeding intolerance Abdominal distention Delayed gastric emptying Bile stained nasogastric tube aspirates Apnea Respiratory distress	Tracheal-esophageal fistula Gastroschisis Omphalocele Necrotizing enterocolitis Intussusception	Circulatory status Fluid resuscitation Reduce risk of dehydration and hypothermia Airway maintenance, Intubation Avoid large tidal volumes Avoid high oxygen concentrations	

Modified Parkland formula for fluid resuscitation: Resuscitation fluids 3–4 mL lactated Ringer solution × weight (kilograms) × %TBSA burned (second degree and third-degree); half administered over the first 8 h (from time of injury), remaining half administered over the next 16 h + maintenance fluids.[11]

Abbreviation: TBSA, total body surface area.

Adapted from McDougall RJ. Paediatric emergencies. Anaesthesia 2013;68(Suppl 1):61–71; and Fabia R. Surgical treatment of burns and management. Medscape. Available at: http://reference.medscape.com/article/934173-treatment. Accessed August 31, 2014.

SUMMARY

Pediatric patients are as unique as their anatomy, physiology, and pathophysiology. A thorough understanding of the pediatric patient is helpful in providing care, especially during emergent situations in the operating room, which can be accomplished by assessing the pediatric patient, dosing medications accurately, and performing effective Pediatric Advanced Life Support. The critical care nurse must also possess a working knowledge of pediatric emergencies, including definition, presentation, pathophysiology, management, and special considerations.

REFERENCES

1. Dieckmann R, Brownstein D, Gausche-Hill M. The pediatric assessment triangle: a novel approach for the rapid evaluation of children. Pediatr Emerg Care 2010; 26(4):312–5.
2. Horeczko T, Enriquez B, McGrath NE, et al. The pediatric assessment triangle: accuracy of its application by nurses in the triage of children. J Emerg Nurs 2013;39(2):182–93.
3. Meguerdichian MJ, Clapper TC. The Broselow tape as an effective medication dosing instrument: a review of the literature. J Pediatr Nurs 2012;27:416–20.
4. Kleinman ME, Chameides L, Schexnayder SM, et al. Pediatric advanced life support: 2010 American Heart Association guidelines for cardiopulmonary resuscitation and emergency cardiovascular care. Pediatrics 2010;126(5):e1361–99.
5. McDougall RJ. Paediatric emergencies. Anaesthesia 2013;68(Suppl 1):61–71.
6. Pitfield AF, Carroll AB, Kissoon N. Emergency management of increased intracranial pressure. Pediatr Emerg Care 2012;28(2):200–4.
7. Stoner MJ, Dulaurier M. Pediatric ENT emergencies. Emerg Med Clin North Am 2013;31(3):795–808.
8. Barata IA. Cardiac emergencies. Emerg Med Clin North Am 2013;31(3):677–704.
9. Choi J, Lee GL. Common pediatric respiratory emergencies. Emerg Med Clin North Am 2012;30(2):529–63.
10. Alalami AA, Ayoub CM, Baraka AS. Laryngospasm: review of different prevention and treatment modalities. Paediatr Anaesth 2008;18(4):281–8.
11. Fabia R. Surgical treatment of burns and management. Medscape Web site. 2014. Available at: http://reference.medscape.com/article/934173-treatment. Accessed August 31, 2014.

APPENDIX 1: PEDIATRIC CARDIAC ARREST

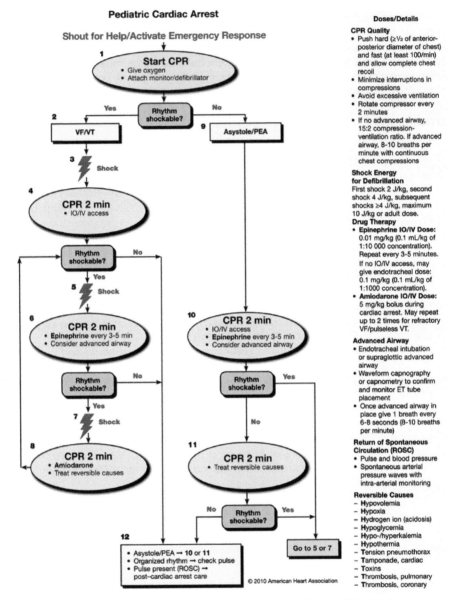

Reprinted with permission from 2010 AHA Guidelines for CPR and ECC. Part 14: Pediatric Advanced Life Support. Circulation 2010;122(suppl 3):S876–908. ©2010 American Heart Association, Inc.

APPENDIX 2: PEDIATRIC BRADYCARDIA

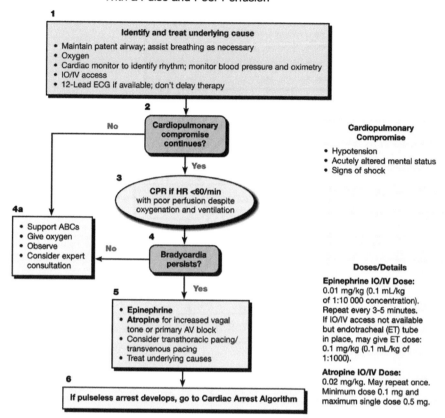

© 2010 American Heart Association

Reprinted with permission from 2010 AHA Guidelines for CPR and ECC. Part 14: Pediatric Advanced Life Support. Circulation 2010;122(suppl 3):S876–908. ©2010 American Heart Association, Inc.

APPENDIX 3: PEDIATRIC TACHYCARDIA

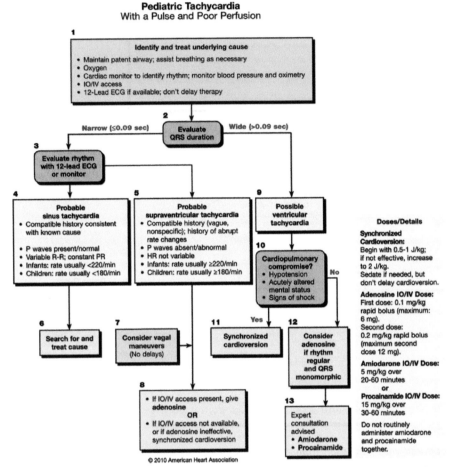

Reprinted with permission from 2010 AHA Guidelines for CPR and ECC. Part 14: Pediatric Advanced Life Support. Circulation 2010;122(suppl 3):S876–908. ©2010 American Heart Association, Inc.

Management of the Patient with Chronic Pain

Renee N. Benfari, BA, MSN, CRNA

KEYWORDS

- Chronic pain • Perioperative • Opioid • Pain • Analgesia

KEY POINTS

- Chronic pain in hospitalized patients remains a challenge in the perioperative setting.
- Despite recent publications and research, no specific guidelines for a multimodal approach to treat patients with chronic pain have been established.
- The preoperative assessment is crucial to evaluate all patients with chronic pain preoperatively.
- Numerous treatment options should be selected and administered based on patients' specific needs.

Chronic pain can be defined as ongoing or recurrent pain, lasting beyond the usual course of an acute illness or injury, which adversely affects the individual's well-being.[1] The International Association for the Study of Pain (IASP) defines chronic pain as a multidimensional phenomenon characterized by unpleasant sensory and emotional experiences.[2] Chronic pain is classified by the pathophysiology as nociceptive or neuropathic, with various or undetermined causes. Neuropathic pain is initiated or caused by a primary lesion or dysfunction in the peripheral or central nervous system.[3] Chronic pain may be associated with cancer, terminal illnesses other than cancer, or chronification of pain.[4] The term chronification of pain is primarily used to describe episodic pain that becomes chronic.[4] By contrast, acute pain is often defined as pain of recent onset, is transient, and elicits a warning that injury or illness has occurred.[5] The duration of chronic pain typically lasts longer than 12 weeks in comparison with acute pain, whose duration is less than 12 weeks.[3]

The management of chronic pain is a complex problem worldwide.[6] Within the perioperative setting it is very common to encounter patients with preexisting chronic pain. According to the National Center for Health Statistics, approximately 25% of the American population has chronic or recurring pain, and 40% report that the pain has a moderate to severe degrading impact on the quality of life. Chronic pain affects more than 70 million patients, and acute pain can lead to chronic pain if not treated properly.[7,8]

Department of Anesthesiology, Yale-New Haven Hospital, 20 York Street, New Haven, CT 06510, USA
E-mail address: Renee.Benfari@YNHH.org

Crit Care Nurs Clin N Am 27 (2015) 121–129
http://dx.doi.org/10.1016/j.cnc.2014.10.001
0899-5885/15/$ – see front matter © 2015 Elsevier Inc. All rights reserved.

According to the Institute of Medicine (IOM) report on pain, chronic pain affects an estimated 116 million American adults and cost the nation up to $635 billion in medical treatment and lost worker productivity.[9] Chronic pain is associated with significant physical, psychological, and social impacts. The concept of managing chronic, noncancerous pain in adults and children has evolved since the early 1980s.[5] Management of chronic pain is frequently complicated by the presence of multiple comorbid conditions, including other disease states, obesity, and mental health disorders.[10] Furthermore, patients with chronic pain do not form a homogeneous group, and include pediatric, adult, and geriatric patients.[4] Sex-based differences in the experience of pain may also create difficulties for the provider of pain management.

Management of chronic pain has created a long-standing problem in the perioperative environment. Poorly managed patients with chronic pain can extend the hospital stay, increase the cost of care, compromise patient satisfaction, and cause suffering.[11] The IOM suggests that major steps need to be taken in the areas of prevention, treatment, education, and research related to the care of patients with pain.[9] The National Center for Health Statistics estimated that in 2006 25% of the American population had chronic or recurring pain. In addition, more than 80% of the 73 million patients undergoing surgery in the United States annually experience postoperative pain and more than 85% of these patients experience moderate, severe, or extreme pain.[11] A multidisciplinary and multimodal approach is essential throughout the perioperative environment to efficiently care for patients with chronic pain.[12]

Pain often occurs in patients under critical care, and is one of the most challenging problems facing nurses in the postoperative environment.[5] In addition to a preexisting chronic pain condition, increases in pain and discomfort can be due to surgical and posttraumatic wounds, invasive monitoring devices, prolonged immobilization, and routine nursing procedures.[5] Strategies for improving pain management practices include providing documentation, implementing pain guidelines, using algorithms, and increasing education in pain management.[13] To provide the best possible care for patients with chronic pain, patient care providers must understand the physiology of pain and its various manifestations.[5] At the Institute for Chronic Pain, the following issues were cited as reasons as to why chronic pain is poorly treated[1]:

- A long-standing and still commonly held view, even among some providers, that chronic pain is the result of a long-lasting acute injury, usually conceived as an orthopedic condition
- A lack of understanding of the role of central sensitization in chronic pain
- Health care provider recommendations that commonly do not follow established clinical guidelines
- A resulting odd state of affairs within the health care system whereby the typical patient with chronic pain obtains the least effective treatments first and obtains the most effective care last
- Third-party reimbursement policies that make the least effective treatments the most profitable to provide and the most effective treatments the least profitable to provide (which may in part lead to the odd state of affairs that patients typically obtain the least effective treatments first)

PAIN IN CHILDREN

Chronic pain is a significant problem is the pediatric population, conservatively estimated to affect 20% to 35% of children and adolescents worldwide.[14,15] According to the American Pain Society, chronic pain in children is a result of a dynamic integration of biological processes, psychological factors, and sociocultural factors considered within a developmental trajectory. This classification of pain includes persistent and recurrent pain in children with chronic health conditions (eg, sickle cell disease or cancer) and pain that is the disorder itself (eg, migraine, functional abdominal pain, complex regional pain syndrome).[5]

The specialty of pediatric pain has undergone a dramatic change since the early 1970s. Pain in children was ignored in health care research because of a few false common practitioner assumptions.[5] The common beliefs were that children did not experience pain because of their immature nervous system, or that they would not remember the pain to the extent that adults do.[5] Furthermore, children were often severely undermedicated or not medicated at all for pain. The changes in pediatric pain management were transformed in the late 1980s as a result of research and legislation to promote the development of drugs for pain.[5] There is now substantial evidence indicating not only that children do experience pain, but also that the pain experience may have long-term chronic pain consequences. Research has confirmed that a lack of analgesia for pain causes "rewiring" in the nerve pathways of pain transmission.[5] However, the misperception that infants have immature nervous systems and do not feel pain remains a common belief.

This myth that children do not experience chronic pain remains at large. Therefore, both the assessment and management of chronic pain in children must be based on the multidimensional pain experience and take into account the contribution of psychological factors, social factors, and biological processes.[14] The evolution of pain treatment in children has documented evidence that not only have children experienced pain but also that the pain experience may have long-term adverse consequences.[5]

PAIN IN THE ELDERLY

The changes in today's aging society will have a major impact on the management of chronic pain in the elderly. Chronic pain is found to diminish the quality of life in the elderly by increasing depression, social isolation, immobility, falls, weight loss, poor appetite, cognitive impairment, and decreased quality of sleep.[15] There will continue to be a dramatic shift from acute to chronic illnesses, making the delivery of adequate health care more complex. Chronic pain in the elderly population is often used interchangeably with the term "persistent pain."[15] The newer term persistent pain is preferred because it is not associated with the negative attitudes and stereotypes that clinicians and patients often associate with the label "chronic pain."[15] Persistent pain or its inadequate treatment is associated with numerous adverse outcomes in older patients, including falls, functional impairment, slow rehabilitation, mood changes, decreased socialization, sleep and appetite disturbances, and greater health care use and costs.[16]

Clinical manifestations of persistent pain are often complex and multifactorial in the older population. In addition, older people often underreport pain.[17] Concurrent illnesses and multiple problems make pain evaluation and treatment more difficult. The treatment method of an average elderly patient will shift to the ongoing management of multiple diseases and disabilities with more than one pharmacologic intervention.[18] Pharmacokinetic and metabolic changes associated with increased age make the elderly vulnerable to side effects and overdosing associated with analgesic agents.[19] Furthermore, altered communication skills, diminished cognitive abilities, or the failure of basic reflexes resulting from aging will alter the reaction to painful events in this population.[5]

The approach to pain management in the elderly differs from that for younger people. Treatment of chronic pain in the elderly must be multidimensional, and includes both noninvasive and invasive therapies.[19] The elderly population is more likely to experience medication-related side effects and have a higher potential for complications and adverse events related to diagnostic and invasive procedures.[20] Perioperative assessments should be thorough in this population to develop the best treatment plan based on the current regimen. Therefore, it is essential for clinicians to understand the impact of chronic pain and effective management in the elderly population.

A patient with chronic pain has certain unique features imperative for perioperative clinicians to obtain preoperatively. The ideal situation for patients with chronic pain is to have a preoperative appointment with the anesthesia team well ahead of surgery.[21] A preanesthesia evaluation is necessary to educate patients, organize resources for preoperative improvement of the patient's physical function, choose optimal anesthetic techniques, and formulate plans for pain management during postoperative recovery.[22]

The era of an increasingly aging population with complex medical problems and chronic pain presents new demands on the perioperative clinician.[23] Anesthesiologists have been trained to treat acute pain, and the need to treat patients with chronic pain intraoperatively has shifted their training and education to addressing an opioid-tolerant population.[11,23] Chronic pain is not the same as acute pain; the pathophysiology and psychological responses to chronic pain are very distinct.[23] Opioid-based analgesia involves potent preparations that confer a high degree of tolerance for patients with chronic pain.[23]

The preoperative evaluation visit must include questions regarding chronic pain and regular use of analgesics and adjuvant medications in addition to signs of psychiatric comorbidity and aberrant drug-related behavior. Altered opioid sensitivity and behavior should also be considered. Moreover, it is essential to document specific details of the underlying pain, such as location, intensity, quality, and relieving factors.[21,22] Preoperative management of opioid-tolerant patients should include their daily maintenance or baseline opioids, and should maintain any transdermal patch they typically use for the day of surgery.[23] Patients who have forgotten their morning medications should be pretreated before the start of the case.

The main objective for the preoperative visit is to help achieve an individualized patient-centered care plan. Clinicians need to be aware that chronic patients may feel frustrated, isolated, angry, or anxious about their surgery if anesthesia does not individualize their perioperative analgesia.[23] Patients with chronic pain are typically managed by multiple providers and have firm beliefs about their chronic pain, and hold high expectations for all clinicians to do the same. The clinician-patient relationship is based on establishing trust by understanding and recognizing chronic pain.[22,23] Patients should feel comfortable in expressing their expectations and concerns with the anesthesia provider. Misconceptions about the surgical procedure, the role of the anesthesiologist in perioperative care, and treatment of postoperative pain are also common in patients. Once a plan for anesthesia is developed, a consultation with the pain service on the day of the procedure should be arranged for most patients with chronic pain.[21]

Patients with chronic pain are often pretreated with opioids, cyclooxygenase inhibitors, antidepressants, anticonvulsants, or any combination of these treatments.[21,22,24] Moreover, they suffer from prolonged inactivity or neurologic deficits (or both), which increases the risk for adverse events during the perioperative period.[22] Tolerance, drug interactions, and side effects may occur. In addition, inappropriate or excessive medication is commonly observed. Patients with chronic pain tend to underestimate and underreport their medication use.[9,22]

Furthermore, analgesic gaps can occur when patients with chronic pain do not take their pain medication on the morning of the surgery and do not inform the anesthesia provider. Both the anesthesia provider and surgeon will ultimately be unable to compensate for the missed doses, and an analgesic gap will occur.[9,22] Thus, under-treatment during the perioperative period may be unnoticed and might induce withdrawal, which can result in serious cardiopulmonary strain associated with the neuroexcitatory withdrawal syndrome.[22,23] In addition, two areas of special concern in opioid-tolerant patients are gastric aspiration and cardiac arrhythmias.[23]

Gastric aspiration is a potentially fatal complication of anesthesia in patients who present with a delay in gastric emptying, decreased gastric motility, and gastric tone or increased pyloric tone.[23] Although the exact mechanism for delay in gastric emptying by opioids is unclear, both central and peripheral mechanisms have been identified.[23] Cardiac arrhythmias represent a significant risk factor for patients undergoing surgery with general anesthesia. Older age, female sex, reduced ejection fraction, left ventricular hypertrophy, ischemia, bradycardia, and electrolyte imbalances have been identified as causative factors in QT prolongation.[23] Furthermore, QT prolongation has been identified in some patients with chronic pain on methadone.[23,25] Therefore, it is essential for anesthesia providers to monitor and provide the safest anesthetic in this high-risk population.

MANAGEMENT OF CHRONIC PAIN

Pain management has become a specialty in the perioperative environment. Perioperative pain control can occur at three specific intervals in relation to surgery: pre-, intra-, and postoperatively.[26] There are numerous methods of analgesic administration for the management of perioperative pain in the patient with chronic pain. Successful pain management entails providing adequate analgesia without excessive adverse side effects.[27]

Specific approaches toward perioperative management of patients with chronic pain are often inadequately described in pain management guidelines.[28] Intraoperative preventive and multimodal analgesia have been introduced to reduce central sensitization, and this has provided an overall benefit in reducing both acute and chronic postoperative pain.[29] Regional anesthesia, adjuvant analgesics, transdermal analgesics, intravenous patient-controlled anesthesia, intravenous/intramuscular medications, local anesthetics, and combination therapy techniques are used in the perioperative setting.[26] Other actions include the administration of preoperative sedatives, administration of nonsteroidal anti-inflammatory drugs, sublingual analgesia, and transcutaneous electrical nerve stimulation.[4,26]

The recent literature provides support for regional anesthesia techniques being superior to opioids alone in the management of pain in patients with chronic pain.[28] The benefits include improved surgical outcomes for thoracic, orthopedic, gynecologic, and general surgery in patients with comorbidities (coexisting chronic pain, morbid obesity, and obstructive sleep apnea).[28] Regional anesthesia has been associated with better patient satisfaction, and results in decreased perioperative morbidity and mortality for patients with comorbid diseases.[28] Another benefit of the use of regional anesthesia is the reduction of opioid-induced hyperalgesia (OIH).[28]

OIH, defined as a state of nociceptive sensitization caused by exposure to opioids,[30,31] is characterized by a paradoxic response whereby a patient receiving opioids for the treatment of pain could actually become more sensitive to certain painful stimuli.[32] The type of pain experienced might be the same as the underlying pain or might be different from the original underlying pain.[32] OIH appears to be a distinct, definable, and characteristic phenomenon that could explain the loss of opioid efficacy in some patients.[11,31] Chronic opioid therapy could paradoxically induce or sensitize patients to acute OIH. Patients on high doses of long-term opioid pharmacotherapy can suffer exquisite acute pain after surgery, creating an escalation in dosing of chronic opioid therapy.[11,31]

Although recent advances have become available for the use of regional anesthesia in the management of patients with chronic pain, many techniques are apparently unexplored and remain underutilized.[28] Other techniques are often used in the intraoperative management of chronic pain.

Ketamine is an N-methyl-D-aspartate (NMDA) receptor antagonist that is used to reduce acute postoperative pain and analgesic consumption in many surgical interventions.[24,32] Ketamine infusions should be considered for patients with opioid tolerance, neuropathic pain, and at risk for developing postoperative pain.[21] The benefits of ketamine include decreasing excitability, decreasing acute postoperative opiate tolerance, and a possible modulation of opiate receptors.[33] Dosing of ketamine for intraoperative infusion varies in both studies and institutions.[21] However, the common regime is to administer an intravenous bolus of 0.25 to 0.5 mg/kg after induction, followed by a continuous infusion of 0.25 to 0.5 mg/kg/h.[21,25] The use of ketamine in a multimodal approach to managing chronic pain provides a reduction in overall opiate consumption.[24,33]

Methadone is an opioid analgesic often used intraoperatively for rapid analgesia if necessary.[25] The NMDA-antagonist properties of methadone have been proved to reduce postoperative opioid requirements by half. A single intravenous dose of methadone (0.2 mg/kg) before surgical incision might be beneficial.[25] However, dosing must be appropriate to the patient's opioid tolerance and or other health comorbidities that could be detrimental. The long half-life and late-peaking respiratory depression of methadone makes dosing extremely important for patients who have obstructive sleep apnea or any pulmonary disease that may reduce ventilatory capacity.[25]

Nonsteroidal anti-inflammatory drugs (NSAIDs) and intravenous acetaminophen have been used as adjuncts to opioid analgesia.[24,25] The site of action of the analgesic effect of acetaminophen is thought to be the central nervous system. Acetaminophen is a synthetic, nonopiate, and antipyretic agent derived from p-aminophenol. The antipyretic effect is thought to be mediated by the inhibition of prostaglandin synthesis within the hypothalamus.[33] The opioid-sparing qualities of acetaminophen have been recognized, and these properties may lead to acetaminophen being incorporated effectively as an adjunctive therapy.[34,35] Intravenous acetaminophen has possible advantages in comparison with intravenous opioid or NSAID analgesia in a variety of orthopedic procedures, including hip fracture repair, adolescent scoliosis surgery, and pediatric hip surgery.[34] Intravenous acetaminophen has no effect on gastrointestinal motility, platelet function and bleeding, renal function, or bone healing, and is not associated with confusion, respiratory depression, or ileus.[34,35]

Anticonvulsants such as gabapentin and pregabalin are often used to treat neuropathic pain.[21,25] These drugs directly reduce the central sensitization of pain by binding to calcium channels, and indirectly inhibit NMDA receptors.[25] In addition, the use of antidepressants is effective in the management of neuropathic pain.[21,25] Medications for neuropathic pain should be continued or increased as necessary in the patient with chronic pain.[21] Recent studies have suggested that gabapentin and pregabalin reduce postoperative morphine requirements and movement pain related to surgery, providing a protective effect that may diminish the hyperalgesia response to surgery.[36]

Other multimodal approaches in the perioperative setting include the use of benzodiazepines, intravenous lidocaine, epidurals, α2-agonists, and local anesthetics.

Anesthesia providers should use and optimize patients' treatment according the surgical procedure and patients' preoperative condition. Intraoperative opioid management by hourly dosing should be established to avoid an analgesic gap.[21] Typically opioid requirements may increase to 30% to 100% over preoperative doses when treating intraoperative acute or chronic pain.[37]

Epidural placement for patients with chronic pain is often promoted for thoracic, abdominal, or bilateral lower leg extremity surgeries.[21] In addition, peripheral nerve blocks with or without indwelling catheters are encouraged for patients with complex pain undergoing extremity surgery.[21] Nerve plexus blocks can provide optimal postoperative analgesia for an extended period of time, decreasing the amount of opioids required.[21]

The initial postoperative period still remains a period of significant undertreatment of pain. Inadequate postoperative pain control following surgery promotes prolonged recovery time, increased morbidity, and decreased satisfaction with care.[11] Barriers within the postoperative setting hinder the improvement of postoperative pain for patients with chronic pain.[11,17] Among the barriers to improving pain control, inadequate clinician knowledge and understanding of therapeutic strategies for pain prevention and control results in inadequate opioid administration.[11]

Another barrier in providing effective postoperative pain management is the provider's tendency to view pain as "expected" rather than acknowledging the needs of a patient with chronic pain.[17] Patients may fear being labeled a complainer, and are often reluctant to report pain to providers.[17,38] Other barriers include the administration of medication and decreased dosing based on gender and racial disparities.[17] Providers often fear overdosing, and may perceive minority patients as having drug-seeking behaviors.[11,17] Therefore, caring for the surgical patient who has a chronic pain condition is a common challenge for the acute pain management clinician in the perioperative environment.[11]

Chronic pain affects approximately 100 million Americans who undergo surgery and experience significant postoperative pain.[9] Providing safe and effective treatment of postoperative pain presents a significant challenge to the perioperative health care team.[9,21] Chronic pain management has been identified as an initiative in the perioperative setting, suggesting that multimodal analgesia can provide an overall reduction in both acute and chronic pain in the perioperative setting.[12] Numerous techniques, medications, and interventions have been identified and are used differently across the United States. Further research and education, and the establishment of guidelines for the treatment of patients with chronic pain in the perioperative environment are imperative to the improvement and delivery of excellent care.

REFERENCES

1. American Chronic Pain Association. Glossary. 2014. Available at: http://www.theacpa.org/glossary. Accessed August 24, 2014.
2. World Health Organization. WHO guidelines on the pharmacological treatment of persisting pain in children with medical illnesses. 2012. Available at: http://www.ncbi.nlm.nih.gov/books/NBK138354/pdf/TOC.pdf. Accessed August 14, 2014.
3. Taverner T, Closs SJ, Briggs M. The journey to chronic pain: a grounded theory of older adults' experiences of pain associated with leg ulceration. Pain Manag Nurs 2014;15(1):186–98.
4. Pergolizzi JV, Taylor R, Muniz E. The role of patient-controlled analgesia in the management of chronic pain. Eur J Pain Suppl 2011;(5):457–63.

5. Helms JE, Barone CP. Physiology and treatment of pain. Crit Care Nurse 2008; 28(6):38–47.
6. Breen J. Transitions in the concept of chronic pain. ANS Adv Nurs Sci 2002;24(4): 48–59.
7. Hasenbring M, Hallner D, Klasen B. Psychological mechanism in the transition from acute to chronic pain: over- or underrated? Schmerz 2001;15:442–7.
8. Katz J, Jackson M, Kavanagh B, et al. Acute pain after thoracic surgery predicts long-term post-thoracotomy pain. Clin J Pain 1996;12(1):50–5.
9. Dykstra KM. Perioperative pain management in the opioid-tolerant patient with chronic pain: an evidence-based practice project. J Perianesth Nurs 2012; 27(6):385–92.
10. Butchart A, Kerr EA, Heisler M, et al. Experience and management of chronic pain among patients with other complex chronic conditions. Clin J Pain 2010; 25(4):293–8.
11. Chapman CR, Davis J, Donaldson GW. Postoperative pain experience: results from a national survey suggest postoperative pain continues to be undermanaged. J Pain 2011;12(12):1240–6.
12. Cho AR, Kwon JY, Kim KH, et al. The effects of anesthetics on chronic pain after breast surgery. Anesth Analg 2013;116(3):685–93.
13. Shannon K, Bucknall T. Pain assessment in critical care: what we have learnt from research. Intensive Crit Care Nurs 2003;19(3):154–62.
14. American Pain Society. Assessment and management of children with chronic pain. 2012. Available at: www.americanpainsociety.org/uploads/pdfs/aps12-pcp.pdf. Accessed August, 2014.
15. Fowler TO, Durham CO, Planton J, et al. Use of nonsteroidal anti-inflammatory drugs in the older adult. J Am Assoc Nurse Pract 2014;26:414–23.
16. The American Geriatric Society. The management of persistent pain in older persons. J Am Geriatr Soc 2002;50:S205–24.
17. Tai-Seale M, Bolin J, Bao X, et al. Management of chronic pain among older patients: inside primary care in the US. Eur J Pain 2011;15:1087.e1–8.
18. Wiener JM, Tilly J. Population ageing in the United States of America: Implications for public programmes. Int J Epidemiol 2002;31:776–81.
19. Vadivelu N, Hines RL. Management of chronic pain in the elderly: focus on transdermal buprenorphine. Bethesda (MD): Dove Medical Press Limited; 2008.
20. The American Geriatric Society. Pharmacological management of persistent pain in older persons. 2009. Available at: http://www.americangeriatrics.org/files/documents/2009_Guideline.pdf. Accessed August 25, 2014.
21. Tumber PS. Optimizing perioperative analgesia for the complex pain patient: medical and interventional strategies. Can J Anaesth 2013;61:131–40.
22. Miller RD. Acute and chronic effects of postoperative pain. In: Miller RD, Fisher LA, Erikkson LI, et al, editors. Miller's anesthesia. Philadelphia: Elsevier Health Sciences; 2009. p. 2757–82.
23. Rozen D, Grass GW. Perioperative and intraoperative pain and anesthetic care of the chronic pain and cancer pain patient receiving chronic opioid therapy. Pain Pract 2005;5(1):18–32.
24. Alencar de Castro R, Leal PC, Sakata RK. Pain management in burn patients. Rev Bras Anestesiol 2012;63(1):149–53.
25. Mueller MF, Golembiewshi J. The changing landscape of perioperative pain management. J Perianesth Nurs 2011;26(4):290–3.
26. Olorunto WA, Galandiuk S. Managing the spectrum of surgical pain: acute management of the chronic pain patient. J Am Coll Surg 2006;202:169–75.

27. Kapur BM, Lala PK, Shaw JL. Pharmacogenetics of chronic pain management. Clin Biochem 2014;47:1169–87.
28. Souzdalnitski D, Halaszynski TM, Faclier G. Regional anesthesia and co-existing chronic pain. Curr Opin Anaesthesiol 2010;23:662–70.
29. Ong CK, Lirk P, Seymour RA, et al. The efficacy of preemptive analgesia for acute postoperative pain management: a meta-analysis. Anesth Analg 2005;100(3): 757–73.
30. Lee M, Silverman S, Hansen H, et al. A comprehensive review of opioid-induced hyperalgesia. Pain Physician 2011;14:145–61.
31. Kim SH, Stoicea N, Soghomonyan S, et al. Intraoperative use of remifentanil and opioid induced hyperalgesia/acute opioid tolerance: systematic review. Front Pharmacol 2014;5(108):1–9.
32. Loftus RW, Yeager MP, Clark JA, et al. Intraoperative ketamine reduces perioperative opiate consumption in opiate-dependent patients with chronic back pain undergoing back surgery. Anesthesiology 2010;113(3):639–46.
33. Graham G, Scott K. Mechanism of action of paracetamol. Am J Ther 2005;12: 46–55.
34. Jahr JS, Lee VK. Intravenous acetaminophen. Anesthesiol Clin 2010;28(4):619–45.
35. Gousheh S, Nesioonour S, Javaher Foroosh F, et al. Intravenous paracetamol for postoperative analgesia in laparoscopic cholecystectomy. Anesth Pain Med 2013;3(1):214–8.
36. Gilron I. Is gabapentin a broad-spectrum analgesic? Anesthesiology 2002;97: 537–9.
37. Mitra S, Sinatra R. Perioperative management of acute pain in the opioid-dependent patient. Anesthesiology 2004;101:212–27.
38. McNeill S. The hidden error of mismanaged pain: a systems approach. J Pain Symptom Manage 2003;28(1):47–58.

Sedation Options for Intubated Intensive Care Unit Patients

 CrossMark

Jennifer Lacoske, CRNA, APRN, MS

KEYWORDS

- Critical care sedation • Analgesia • Agitation • Delirium • Intensive care • Protocols
- Sedation infusions

KEY POINTS

- Targeted light sedation and daily interruption protocols are the preferred methods for sedation administration in the intensive care unit.
- Assessment of pain, agitation, and delirium is an integrated process, which should guide pharmacologic and nonpharmacologic interventions in the patient's plan of care.
- When administering procedural sedation, understanding the scope of practice and limits of medication dosing for an individual's scope of practice can help optimize patient safety and prevent adverse events.

WHY WE SEDATE

The intubated intensive care unit (ICU) patient requires a complex care regimen, addressing both physiologic and psychological needs. A patient requiring an endotracheal tube for mechanical ventilation may be difficult to manage. Often, patients are sedated for overall comfort and safety. Numerous studies have been conducted to determine the best regimen for optimized patient outcomes when using different sedation protocols. These studies have explored both optimal sedation medication combinations and protocols for weaning to a timely and successful extubation. In this article, the reasons we sedate, measures of sedation and pain assessment, suggestions for tapering sedation, and the individual medications commonly prescribed to maintain sedation for the intubated ICU patient are discussed. The topic of procedural sedation for the ICU patient in the out of unit setting is also explored.

PAIN, SEDATION, AND DELIRIUM ASSESSMENT

Part of everyday practice in the intensive care setting is a daily and ongoing assessment of pain, sedation, and delirium. The Society of Critical Care Medicine's (SCCM)

No disclosures to report.
Department of Anesthesiology, Yale-New Haven Hospital, 20 York Street, New Haven, CT 06510, USA
E-mail address: jlacoske@yahoo.com

Crit Care Nurs Clin N Am 27 (2015) 131–145
http://dx.doi.org/10.1016/j.cnc.2014.10.006
0899-5885/15/$ – see front matter © 2015 Elsevier Inc. All rights reserved.

2013 *Clinical Practice Guidelines for the Management of Pain, Agitation, and Delirium in Critically Ill Patients* are heavily referenced throughout this article to provide the standards for management of this type of patient in the ICU. The guidelines are based on systematic review of the literature and evidence-based practice. These guidelines were revised from the originals published in 2002, which directed the sustained use of sedatives and analgesics in the critically ill patient. The guidelines are intended to provide a roadmap for developing integrated, evidence-based, and patient-centered protocols for preventing, assessing, and managing pain, agitation, and delirium in the critically ill patient.[1] A combination of narcotics and benzodiazepines is most commonly used to sedate intubated patients. To properly tailor a drug regimen to the patient, one must understand how to assess patient needs.

All patients, regardless of the specialty of the ICU, or the severity of patient condition, can experience routine pain and discomfort related to ICU care, even while at rest.[1] A negative psychological outcome of prolonged pain exposure in the ICU is posttraumatic stress disorder (PTSD). Although most studies have found the incidence of PTSD to be low in patients living after an ICU stay, a range of 18% to 27% were still found to have this experience.[1–3] Pain has been found to be responsible for numerous adverse physiologic responses, including unstable hemodynamics, hyperglycemia, alterations of immune system function, and increase in catecholamine, cortisol, and antidiuretic hormone levels.[4,5] Increased catecholamines lead to arteriolar vasoconstriction, resulting in impairment of tissue oxygenation.[1,6] Catabolic stimulation and hypoxemia significantly impair wound healing and increase the risk of wound infection.[1] Pain also suppresses natural killer cell activity by decreasing cytotoxic T cells and reduction of neutrophil phagocytic activity, resulting in critical impairment of the immune system.[1,7,8] All of these physiologic factors can lead to worsening of patient condition, increase in complications, and prolonged length of stay for the patient.

The gold standard of pain assessment is a self-report. When a patient cannot self-report pain, an assessment tool must be used for determining pain measurement. The standard scales for pain assessment in a patient unable to self-report pain as determined by the SCCM are the Behavioral Pain Scale (BPS) and the Critical Care Pain Observation Tool (CPOT). Despite being the standard for pain measurement, the scales are limited for patients with chronic pain and delirium, as well as patients who are incapable of neuromuscular movements.[4] **Table 1** provides an example of a combination of scales used for patient assessment to give a general idea of the type of measures that all of the nonverbal pain scales use. Although there are many different scales to assess pain, with similar parameters assessed, the CPOT has been proved to have the highest reliability, followed by the BPS.[1,4]

Sedation is provided to intubated patients for several reasons. The most common reason is for anxiety. Anxiety is defined as a sustained state of apprehension and autonomic arousal in response to real or perceived threats.[9] Signs and symptoms commonly associated with anxiety include headache, nausea, insomnia, anorexia, dyspnea, palpitations, dizziness, dry mouth, chest pain, diaphoresis, hyperventilation, pallor, tachycardia, tremors, and hypervigilance.[9] Given the physiologic responses to anxiety as listed earlier, it is clear that anxiety has a significant impact on weaning a patient with an endotracheal tube. An absolute indication for pharmacologic sedation is neuromuscular paralysis. It is critical to avoid undue anxiety, awareness, and pain when a patient's condition is fragile enough to require paralysis as part of their plan of care.

The standard assessment tool for monitoring sedation and agitation is the Richmond Agitation-Sedation Scale (RASS) (**Table 2**). Previously, the Ramsay Scale had

Table 1
Nonverbal critical care BPS

Indicator	Descriptives		
Facial Expression	Relaxed without tension	Muscle tension, grimace, frown, brow lowering	Almost constant tension of all muscles, eyes tightly closed
Score	0	1	2
Restlessness/ agitation	Quiet, relaxed, little movement	Occasional movement, shifting, rubs pain site	Frequently restless, pulls at tubes, thrashing, no command following
Score	0	1	2
Muscle tone	Normal tone, without resistance to passive movement	Increased tone with resistance to passive movement	Rigid tone with strong resistance to passive movement
Score	0	1	2
Ventilator compliance (intubated)	Tolerating ventilator without alarming	Cough, occasional alarm not requiring attention	Fighting ventilator, out of synch with modes, frequent alarms requiring intervention
Score	0	1	2
OR			
Vocalization (not intubated)	Normal sounds, talking	Occasional moans, sighs, grunts	Frequent to continuous crying, moaning, sobbing
Score	0	1	2
Consolability	Content, no needs	Reassured by talk, easy to distract	Difficult to comfort by talk or touch
Score	0	1	2

Total score for each category determines pain score: 0, no pain; 1–3, mild pain; 4–6, moderate pain; ≥6, severe pain.

Adapted from Stites M. Observational pain scales in critically ill adults. Crit Care Nurse 2013;33(3):68–78; and Behavioral Pain Scale (nonverbal) for patients unable to provide a self-report of pain. Available at: http://magazine.nursing.jhu.edu/wp-content/uploads/2010/08/PainScale.jpg. Accessed August 12, 2014.

been used to provide measures of sedation and agitation, but higher reliability has been proved with the RASS scale.[10] The SCCM does not recommend objective measures of brain function such as the Bispectral Index or state entropy in patients who are noncomatose or nonparalyzed, because they are inadequate substitutes for subjective sedation scores. However, these objective measures can be used to measure sedation assessment when patients are receiving neuromuscular blocking agents, because patients are unable to be assessed under the RASS scale secondary to inability to initiate spontaneous movements.[1]

Delirium is an important issue to assess for in ICU patients, because it can often be mistaken as anxiety. Delirium has been found to be associated with increased mortality and prolonged ICU and hospital length of stay, as well as development of post-ICU cognitive impairment.[1] Four risk factors significantly associated with the development of delirium are preexisting dementia, history of hypertension, history of alcoholism,

Table 2		
The RASS		
Score	Term	Description
+4	Combative	Overtly combative, violent, immediate danger to staff
+3	Very agitated	Pulls or removes tube(s) or catheter(s); aggressive
+2	Agitated	Frequent nonpurposeful movement, fights ventilator
+1	Restless	Anxious but movements not aggressive vigorous
0	Alert and calm	
−1	Drowsy	Not fully alert, but has sustained awakening (eye opening/eye contact) to voice ($\geq$10 s)
−2	Light sedation	Briefly awakens with eye contact to voice (<10 s)
−3	Moderate sedation	Movement or eye opening to voice (but no eye contact)
−4	Deep sedation	No response to voice, but movement or eye opening
−5	Unarousable	No response to voice or physical stimulation

From Sessler CN, Gosnell M, Grap MJ, et al. The Richmond Agitation-Sedation Scale: validity and reliability in adult intensive care patients. Am J Respir Crit Care Med 2002;166:1338–44; with permission. Copyright © 2002, American Thoracic Society.

and a high severity of illness at ICU admission.[1] Delirium assessments should be conducted on a daily basis as appropriate to patient condition. The Confusion Assessment Method (CAM) for the ICU is the standard assessment tool for the measurement of delirium in the ICU patient (**Table 3**).

Although the focus of this article is pharmacologic interventions, pharmacologic intervention alone is not the only method available to manage patient needs while intubated in the ICU. Later in this article, targeted light sedation and daily interruption protocols are explored, but no pharmacologic standard recommendations are supported for the treatment of delirium. Haloperidol had previously been recommended for use in treatment of delirium, but it is no longer recommended, because of lack of adequate supportive evidence; nor are other antipsychotic agents recommended.[1,11] Early detection of delirium, combined with prevention and nonexacerbating interventions such as early weaning, less use of restraint devices, attempts to normalize sleep-wake patterns, and early mobilization, all help prevent, treat, and decrease duration of delirium.[1] Pain and sedation medications should be tailored to optimize these critical needs of the patient, with the goal of management and prevention of delirium.

MEDICATIONS FOR SEDATION AND ANALGESIA

Common medications used to provide sedation and analgesia to the ICU population are midazolam, lorazepam, dexmedetomidine, propofol, fentanyl, morphine, and hydromorphone. Any combination of these drugs can be administered to provide sedation appropriately tailored to the patient's condition. Most often a combination of benzodiazepine and narcotic infusions is used to maintain sedation and comfort in the ICU setting. Depending on patient condition, the newer SCCM guidelines are moving away from benzodiazepines and favoring shorter-acting infusions, such as propofol and dexmedetomidine, to facilitate timely extubation and decrease risk of delirium. However, these 2 medications are limited, in that they are not recommended for long-term (several day) infusions. **Table 4** provides a reference of the dosing for ICU sedation of the medications to be discussed in this section.

Table 3
CAM-ICU worksheet

	Score	Check If Present
Feature 1: Acute Onset or Fluctuating Course		
Is the patient different than his or her baseline mental status? OR Has the patient had any fluctuations in mental status in the past 24 h as evidenced by fluctuation on a sedation scale (RASS), GCS, or previous delirium assessment?	Either question Yes →	☐
Feature 2: Inattention		
Letters Attention Test Directions: Say to the patient, "I am going to read you a series of 10 letters. Whenever you hear the letter A indicate by squeezing my hand." Read letters from the following letter list in a normal tone 3 s apart S A V E A H A A R T Errors are counted when the patient fails to squeeze on the letter A and when the patient squeezes any other letter than A.	Number of errors >2 →	☐
Feature 3: Altered Level of Consciousness		
Present if the actual RASS score is anything other than alert and calm (zero)	RASS anything other than zero →	☐
Feature 4: Disorganized Thinking		
Yes/No Questions 1. Will a stone float on water? 2. Are there fish in the sea? 3. Does 1 pound weigh more than 2 pounds? 4. Can you use a hammer to pound a nail? Errors are counted when the patient incorrectly answers a question. Command: Say to the patient: "Hold up this many fingers" (Hold 2 fingers in front of the patient) "Now do the same thing with the other hand" (Do not repeat number of fingers) Error is counted if patient is unable to complete the entire command.	Combined number of errors >1 →	☐
Overall CAM-ICU Feature 1 *plus* 2 *and* 3 *or* 4 = **CAM-ICU positive**	Criteria met → Criteria not met →	☐ CAM-ICU Positive (delirium present) ☐ CAM-ICU Negative (no delirium)

Abbreviation: GCS, Glasgow Coma Scale.

Morphine

Morphine sulfate is an opioid agonist relatively selective for the μ receptor in the central nervous system (CNS), although when administered at higher doses, morphine can interact with additional opioid receptors. Pharmacologic effects of all opioid agonists include anxiolysis, euphoria, the feeling of relaxation, cough suppression, and analgesia.[1] The major clearance pathway of morphine is hepatic glucuronidation, which can yield active morphine-6-glucoronide metabolites. Morphine is highly metabolized on first-pass biotransformation, and 90% of metabolites are excreted through the kidneys. The elimination half-life ranges typically from 2.1 to 2.6 hours. Peak analgesia after intravenous (IV) administration occurs after 20 minutes, with duration of analgesia lasting 3 to 6 hours. Maximal respiratory depression is noted at 30 minutes after administration.[12] The active metabolites can be problematic for the elderly with decreased renal and liver function and can lead to greater incidences of delirium, as well as delayed onset of respiratory depression, because of variations in pharmacokinetics secondary to end-organ dysfunction. Guidelines for dosing of morphine in the ICU suggest intermittent dosing of 2 to 4 mg every 1 to 2 hours and infusion rates of 2 to 30 mg/h.[1] Higher doses are often consistent with infusions for the opioid tolerant as well as for end-of-life care.

Morphine has more effects on ancillary organ systems than other opioids, such as fentanyl and hydromorphone. Morphine often causes constipation by slowing gastrointestinal motility and decreasing propulsive contractions of the smooth muscle in the gastrointestinal tract. The biliary tract is also affected, which can lead to worsening pain in patients with biliary colic.[12] In regards to the urinary system, morphine increases tone of the urinary smooth muscle, which can lead to difficulty voiding. Antidiuretic hormone can also be increased, leading to decreased urinary output.[12]

A histamine release is associated with morphine, which can result in the formation of skin wheals and urticaria at the injection site. More severe reactions result in cutaneous vasodilation, causing flushing of the face and neck, along with pruritus and sweating.[12] Depending on the degree of vasodilation, patients may also become nauseated during this experience. Morphine does have effects on the chemoreceptor trigger zone, which can cause nausea and vomiting when stimulated; however,

Table 4
Quick dosing reference table

Medication	IV Infusion Rates	Intermittent Dosing
Morphine	2–30 mg/h	2–4 mg IV every 1–2 h
Hydromorphone	0.5–3 mg/h	0.2–0.6 mg IV every 1–2 h
Fentanyl	0.7–10 µg/kg/h	0.35–0.5 µg/kg IV every 0.5–1 h

Medication	IV Infusion Rates	Loading Doses
Midazolam	0.02–0.1 mg/kg/h	0.01–0.05 mg/kg over several min
Lorazepam	0.01–0.1 mg/kg/h ($\leq$10 mg/h) or 0.02–0.06 mg/kg every 2–6 h as needed	0.02–0.04 mg/kg ($\leq$2 mg)
Propofol	5–50 µg/kg/min no boluses	5 µg/kg/min over 5 min
Dexmedetomidine	0.2–0.7 µg/kg/h	1 µg/kg over 10 min

Adapted from Barr J, Gilles LF, Puntillo K, et al. Clinical practice guidelines for the management of pain, agitation, and delirium in adult patients in the intensive care unit. Crit Care Med 2013;41(1):263–30.

morphine depresses the vomiting center. Thus, subsequent dosing is less likely to cause vomiting once this center has been depressed.[12]

Significant respiratory depression can occur with morphine, making patients with poor respiratory reserve undesirable candidates for its administration. Morphine administration can also result in severe hypotension in patients already experiencing hemodynamic instability or poor fluid volume status.[12] These are important considerations in selecting morphine as part of sedation regimen in the ICU, because the patient condition should always be first and foremost in the mind of the prescriber and the vigilant bedside nurse.

Hydromorphone (Dilaudid)

Hydromorphone is an opioid agonist selective for the μ receptor, with a principal therapeutic action of analgesia. Like morphine and all other opioids, respiratory depression remains a paramount concern, because all of these drugs reduce the responsiveness of the brain stem respiratory center to an increase in carbon dioxide tension.[13] Much like morphine, hydromorphone can cause a decrease in gastric, biliary, and pancreatic secretion, along with decreased motility of the smooth muscle and potential for spasm in the sphincter of Oddi.[13] Traditionally, less histamine release is noted with hydromorphone compared with morphine.

Hydromorphone is extensively metabolized via glucuronidation in the liver to inactive metabolites. Systemic clearance is 1.96 L/min, resulting in a terminal elimination half-life of 2.3 hours after a single IV dose. It is recommended that patients with hepatic impairment be administered one-quarter to one-half the dosing of a nonimpaired patient as well as those patients with renal impairment.[13] The onset of action in the average patient is 5 to 15 minutes from an IV dose. Guidelines for dosing suggest an infusion rate of 0.5 to 3 mg/h for the ICU.[1]

Fentanyl

Fentanyl citrate is a potent opioid agonist with a standard IV dose of 100 μg providing the analgesic equivalent of 10 mg of morphine. Fentanyl has a 3-compartment pharmacokinetic profile, with distribution taking 1.7 minutes, redistribution taking 13 minutes, and a terminal elimination half-time of 219 minutes. The volume of distribution is 4 L/kg, and plasma protein binding increases with increased ionization of the drug. Fentanyl is primarily transformed in the liver, with a high first-pass clearance.[14]

The onset of action of the drug is almost immediate, but the maximal respiratory depressant and analgesic effects may not be noted for several minutes. The usual duration of action of a 1-time, 100-μg dose is 30 to 60 minutes; however, the respiratory depressant effects may outlast the duration of the analgesic effect. The peak respiratory effect is noted 5 to 15 minutes after administration of a single injection. However, decreased sensitivity to CO_2 stimulation can persist longer than the depression of respiratory rate associated with a single dose.[14] This is an important consideration when selecting pain medications, especially as the patient undergoes spontaneous breathing trials (SBTs) close to meeting criteria for extubation.

Because of the significant respiratory effects, the primary indication for fentanyl administration is listed for the operative encounter, because it should be administered only by trained personnel in a monitored setting. Thus, the SCCM has created guidelines for unlabeled dosing, specifically for critically ill patients in an ICU. Those without mechanical ventilation may receive a slow IV bolus of 25 to 35 μg (based on an ideal body weight of 70 kg) or 0.35 to 0.5 μg/kg every 30 to 60 minutes. Continuous IV infusions may be instituted for mechanically ventilated patients with doses ranging from 50 to 700 μg/h or 0.7 to 10 μg/kg/h.[1,15]

Respiratory depression, apnea, chest wall rigidity, and bradycardia are the serious adverse reactions associated with fentanyl, which can lead to respiratory arrest and circulatory depression and result in cardiac arrest. Hypertension, hypotension, dizziness, blurred vision, nausea, emesis, laryngospasm, and diaphoresis may also occur. Precautions should be taken in patients with chronic obstructive pulmonary disease, low respiratory reserve, impaired hepatic and renal function, and cardiac bradyarrhythmias, because these conditions can all be exacerbated by fentanyl administration.[14]

Midazolam (Versed)

Midazolam is a short-acting benzodiazepine with amnestic, anxiolytic, sedative, and hypnotic effects.[1] Benzodiazepines also possess anticonvulsant effects. Sedation is achieved within 3 to 5 minutes of IV injection when the drug acts on the γ-aminobutyric acid A (GABA$_A$) receptors of the CNS. The drug is metabolized by the liver via the cytochrome P450-34A enzyme, thus allowing for increased drug concentrations when this enzyme is inhibited by other medications.[16] Active metabolites are produced as this drug is processed, which presents a problem for those with renal insufficiency.[1,17] The volume of distribution is 1 to 3.1 L/kg and the elimination half-life is 1.8 to 6.4 hours. Women, the elderly, and the obese have higher volumes of distribution. Those with congestive heart failure, hepatic insufficiency, and renal failure have the potential for a greater than 2-fold increase in elimination half-life.[16] Midazolam also crosses the placenta into fetal circulation and can cause an increased risk of congenital malformations in early stages of pregnancy. There is also a contraindication for patients with narrow angle glaucoma.[16]

Serious warnings are listed for administration in a setting without appropriate monitoring and personnel trained to handle airway rescue if an endotracheal tube is not in place. Hypoventilation and airway obstruction are common after administration; if these conditions are left untreated or unrecognized, cardiac arrest can result. There is a cumulative effect when using other CNS depressants such as barbiturates, alcohol, and narcotics with midazolam, resulting in an increase in the risk of respiratory compromise, secondary to additional respiratory depression.[16] Benzodiazepine-induced cardiopulmonary instability is more likely to occur in critically ill patients with existing respiratory insufficiency or cardiovascular instability, because systemic hypotension can result.[1,18] Guidelines for the use of midazolam for sedation of the intubated patient include a loading dose of 0.01 to 0.05 mg/kg over several minutes, followed by dosing of 0.02 to 0.1 mg/kg/h.[1]

Lorazepam (Ativan)

Lorazepam is another benzodiazepine that works by inhibiting the GABA$_A$ receptors of the CNS. Lorazepam is less lipid soluble than midazolam, resulting in a slower uptake and an onset time of 15 to 20 minutes after a loading dose.[1] Metabolism of lorazepam is similar to midazolam, also producing active metabolites, which remain problematic for patients with renal dysfunction.

Most considerations remain the same for lorazepam as for midazolam, because they both act on the same receptor in the CNS with similar effects. Respiratory depression remains a serious concern in the nonintubated patient on initiation of sedation infusions. A loading dose of 0.02 to 0.04 mg/kg over 2 minutes is recommended for initiation, and a maintenance infusion should be dosed at 0.01 to 0.1 mg/kg/h. Bolus dosing as needed of 0.02 to 0.06 mg/kg every 2 to 6 hours may be effective for maintenance as well.[1]

A unique consideration for lorazepam that can limit its usage as the primary sedative in the ICU is its formulation with propylene glycol. Propylene glycol can lead to toxicity, which presents as a metabolic acidosis or an acute kidney injury.[1,19] Dosing as low as 1 mg/kg has been shown to have the potential for toxicity; it was previously believed that only doses of 15 to 25 mg/h could yield such a result.[1,20]

Propofol (Diprivan)

Propofol is a potent sedative, which like most anesthetic agents has a poorly understood mechanism of action, but it is believed to have sedative and hypnotic effects attributed to its action on the $GABA_A$ receptors in the CNS. Additional effects of propofol are anxiolytic, amnestic, antiemetic, and also anticonvulsant.[1] Propofol has a highly lipid-soluble composition, which allows it to rapidly cross the blood-brain barrier and also redistribute into peripheral tissues, thus, allowing for an onset time of 40 seconds to 3 minutes.[1,21] Propofol has a high hepatic clearance, when it is conjugated into inactive metabolites, and thus, when combined with a rapid redistribution, this allows clearance ranges of 1.6 to 3.4 L/min in adults for short-term infusions. Although this quick distribution and elimination profile sounds favorable, as the duration of infusion increases, the steady-state volume of distribution increases. As tissues become saturated, it is possible that a 10-day infusion can reach a distribution of 60 L/kg, which have a terminal half-life of 1 to 3 days. Chronic hepatic cirrhosis and chronic renal impairment do not alter the pharmacokinetics of propofol.[21]

Propofol commonly causes respiratory depression and hypotension secondary to systemic vasodilation. Rapid IV push may result in apnea and profound hypotension and is not recommended to be administered by anyone other than trained anesthesia personnel when an endotracheal tube is not in place. The SCCM recommends ICU sedation dosing for the intubated patient to include a loading dose of 5 μg/kg/min over 5 minutes, followed by a maintenance infusion of 5 to 50 μg/kg/min.[1]

Propofol is an excellent option for units such as the neuro-ICU when the patient has an acute head injury and requires sedation but also needs to be awoken frequently for neurologic assessments. However, infusion is not recommended for more than a few days, because the quick on-off effect diminishes as number of days on infusion increases.

There are other side effects of propofol that deter prescribers from continuing long-term infusions. Hypertriglyceridemia, acute pancreatitis, and myoclonus all have been associated with administration. A rare infusion syndrome, propofol infusion syndrome (PRIS), has been associated typically with prolonged infusion of greater than 70 μg/kg/min.[1] The major signs and symptoms of PRIS include hypertriglyceridemia, worsening metabolic acidosis, and hypotension, with increasing vasopressor requirements as well as arrhythmias. Other associated problems include acute kidney injury, hyperkalemia, rhabdomyolysis, and liver dysfunction.[1,22,23]

Further nursing considerations should involve an allergy assessment, because propofol is contraindicated in patients with allergies to eggs, egg products, soybeans, or soy products. Life-threatening anaphylactic and anaphylactoid reactions are highly likely in patients with these allergies. Also, it is advised that strict aseptic technique be used when handling propofol. Propofol is prepared with 0.005% disodium edentate, which prevents microbial growth for only up to 12 hours.[21] Because of this factor, infusion tubing requires changing every 12 hours.

Dexmedetomidine (Precedex)

Dexmedetomidine is a highly selective α_2-adrenergic agonist possessing sedative properties, which, is indicated for sedation of intubated and mechanically ventilated patients. After administration there is a rapid distribution phase, with a distribution half-life of 6 minutes and a terminal elimination half-life of 2 hours. There is little variability in pharmacokinetic profile for infusions running greater than or less than 24 hours. Dexmedetomidine undergoes biotransformation via direct glucuronidation as well as cytochrome P450-CYP2A6–mediated metabolism. Dosing should be decreased in patients with hepatic impairment. Dosing is recommended as an initial load of 1 μg/kg over 10 minutes, followed by an infusion at 0.2 to 0.7 μg/kg/h.[24]

Major side effects of dexmedetomidine infusion are hypotension, bradycardia, and sinus arrest. Bradycardia and sinus arrest are more prominent in those with high vagal tone. Anticholinergic medications (glycopyrrolate, atropine) may be used to modify vagal tone as an effective treatment of severe bradycardia secondary to infusion. Rapid IV boluses of dexmedetomidine are poorly tolerated and not advised. Patients with preexisting hemodynamic compromise may have profound hypotension with the initial bolus load. The infusion is still highly effective without the bolus load, but the steady state takes longer to achieve. In some cases, the bolus load has been found to cause a transient hypertension as well.[24]

Dexmedetomidine is gaining favorability for weaning patients from mechanical ventilation, as it is the only sedative that does not significantly affect the respiratory drive. Because it does not directly depress the respiratory centers, dexmedetomidine can be continued during extubation to provide comfort to patients throughout the transition. These patients still require an ICU level of monitoring if the infusion is continued after extubation, because hypoventilation and hypoxemia are still possible secondary to loss of oropharyngeal muscle tone.[1,25]

Patients on dexmedetomidine infusions are generally more easily aroused and interactive than those on benzodiazepine or narcotic infusions. Dexmedetomidine seems to reduce requirements of narcotics by the potentiating effects of α_2 agonists. A recent study[1,26] suggested that patients on dexmedetomidine may have a lower prevalence of delirium than patients sedated with midazolam. Future research could yield a preference for dexmedetomidine as a frontline sedative for these many desired effects. There is also a case report[27] using dexmedetomidine to wean a highly addicted patient from both the ventilator and polysubstance abuse with minimal withdrawal side effects. However, this case report used the infusion for 7 days, not the current 24-hour recommendation.

Reversal Agents

Whenever administering medications to a patient, the patient's condition should always be taken into consideration. A patient's response to medication is dependent on a myriad of factors; age, weight, underlying comorbidities, nutritional status, fluid volume status, and ability to mount a stress response all greatly influence how a patient may handle a medication. In the event of a narcotic oversedation, or other undesired side effects, naloxone (Narcan) may be administered. When oversedation or unwanted side effects occur with benzodiazepine administration, flumazenil (Romazicon) may be administered. In the case of an intubated patient in the ICU, these medications are rarely administered. The patient's airway is protected and the patient may be mechanically ventilated until the respiratory depressant effects of the offending drug have dissipated.

When a patient is on a longer duration infusion of sedation, a 1-time dose of reversal is not enough to completely reverse all of the medication in the system, because most medications redistribute into peripheral tissues and take time to process once accumulated. A 1-time dose of reversal is helpful if it is suspected that a bolus of sedative may have caused an acute change in mental status, but overall, time is the only way to completely rid the body of these medications once a steady-state level has been established. The consequences of reversing a narcotic or benzodiazepine must be taken into consideration as well. Patients may become severely agitated and show symptoms of withdrawal when these reversal agents are administered. There are no reversal agents for propofol or dexmedetomidine, because these are neither narcotic nor benzodiazepine medications.

Flumazenil can be used to reverse benzodiazepines per the following dosing[28]: an initial dose of 0.2 mg IV is given over 15 seconds, and repeated doses may be given until a desired level of consciousness is obtained. Repeat doses of 0.2 mg may be repeated at 1-minute intervals until the maximum total cumulative dose of 1 mg is achieved. This dose should not be exceeded. When resedation occurs, repeated doses may be administered at 20-minute intervals per the protocol previously listed. The amount of flumazenil given in a 1-hour period should not exceed 3 mg.

Naloxone can be used to reverse opioids per the following dosage[29]: if an opioid overdose requires advanced cardiac life support, the standard dose of 0.2 to 2 mg IV, intramuscularly, or subcutaneously every 2 to 3 minutes should be administered. The patient likely requires redosing at 20-minute to 60-minute intervals, depending on the type of opioid. If there is respiratory depression associated with therapeutic opioid doses, an initial dose of 0.04 to 0.4 mg may be used to achieve the desired response. After a dose of up to 0.8 mg, other causes of respiratory depression should be considered.[29,30]

Naloxone also has interesting off-label use. It may be given as an infusion at 0.25 μg/kg/h to reduce the side effects of opioid-induced pruritus.[29,31] This method may be helpful in preventing agitation associated with this opioid side effect when using a narcotic infusion as part of sedation/pain management regimen. Often, naloxone is administered in conjunction with neuraxial anesthesia with intrathecal or epidural narcotics, because the pruritus side effect is greater when narcotics are administered by these routes rather than IV or orally.

EFFECTIVE SEDATION AND ANALGESIA WEANING TO EXTUBATION

Patient safety and comfort, along with facilitation of the healing process, are the primary goals of an effective sedation/pain management regimen for the intubated ICU patient. Use of assessment tools can help taper medications in a timely fashion to facilitate the goal of a timely and successful extubation. Many studies have been conducted to ascertain the best way to titrate off medications to facilitate weaning and extubation. The idea of a daily interruption to facilitate spontaneous awakening trials and SBTs has been heavily investigated.

A typical daily interruption protocol involves stopping sedation for a specified period to allow the patient to awaken and perform an SBT. After the trial, the goal is typically to reduce the sedative in half, as mechanical ventilation efforts and overall patient status permit. If appropriate to patient condition, a discontinuation of continuous sedation is preferable if the patient can be maintained by implementing an as-needed dosing plan.

All recent research supports the idea of a light sedation model over a deep sedation model for improved patient outcomes and fewer days of ventilator dependence. One of the earliest randomized controlled trials up for review[32] stated that daily interruption significantly decreases the length of stay in the ICU, however, it did not result in an overall decrease in total length of hospital stay. A follow-up randomized control trial published 8 years later[33] further supported this methodology, stating that interruption trials improved mortality and facilitated decreased length of stay in the ICU as a direct result of patients having fewer days dependent on mechanical ventilation. This study raised concerns over the rate of self-extubation and increased workload on nursing staff when using this type of protocol.

A study[34] involving a multidisciplinary survey to perceived barriers to implementing sedation protocols and daily interruption models was reported shortly after these findings. The top 4 barriers to any protocol were listed to be: increased device removal, poor nursing acceptance, compromise of patient comfort, and a higher incidence of respiratory compromise. No direct recommendations were made to reduce barriers other than to address them on an institutional level to increase acceptance across all disciplines.

A meta-analysis of randomized controlled trials for daily sedation interruption published in 2011[35] suggested that when analyzing all available data, which were stated as limited, there was no significant reduction in duration of mechanical ventilation, length of hospital stay, ICU stay, or mortality associated with a daily interruption model. A need for long-term survival follow-up studies was recommended, because data do not support the practice of daily sedation interruption as superior to any other method.

A more recent study analyzed the daily interruption versus targeted sedation protocols, when sedation was directed by bedside ICU staff rather than a researcher. The thought was that this method would improve practicality and tailor the protocol more accurately to patient needs as assessed by staff. This study tested for the time to a successful extubation and did not find improved outcomes with daily sedative interruption. There was an overall increase in opioid and benzodiazepine administration, as well as a higher self-assessed nursing workload than in the targeted light sedation control group.[36] This finding contradicts earlier claims that the daily interruption protocols resulted in an overall decrease in the total amount of narcotics and benzodiazepines administered.

More recent studies[37] continue to support the idea that deep sedation is suboptimal to improving patient outcome, but there is no supportive evidence to suggest that targeted light sedation models versus daily interruption models have any significantly better outcome, but both are significantly better than a deep sedation model. The SCCM guidelines confirm these findings in their lack of recommendation for either methodology being superior and again shift focus on the continuum of patient assessment for pain, agitation, and delirium to integrate nonpharmacologic-based and pharmacologic-based protocols to improve patient safety and outcomes.[1,37] The SCCM calls for further studies based on long-term outcomes rather than solely the measure of successful extubation or quantity of medication administered, to prove superiority of 1 method over another. However, because these models both follow the principles of lighter sedation, it can only be assumed that with expert assessment skills, what is best for the patient is a patient-centered care plan, which may use either of these techniques.

THE INTENSIVE CARE UNIT REGISTERED NURSE AND PATIENT PROCEDURES

As medicine advances and the ICU acuity increases, patient care is in a constant state of evolution. Although the operating room (OR) was previously the primary site of intervention for patient ailments, advances in medicine have allowed for an explosion of growth for procedural care that can be performed outside the OR. Medical management has gained popularity over surgery for a myriad of conditions that at one time could be managed only from a surgical standpoint. There are a multitude of locations where the ICU registered nurse (RN) may be called on to provide sedation outside the surgical arena. MRI and computed tomography (CT) suites are locations where nurses transport intubated patients and maintain sedation to facilitate imaging. The electrophysiology, gastroenterology, and interventional radiology suites are common for nurse-administered sedation to facilitate procedures as well.

In the OR, maintenance of the patient condition and anesthetic depth are typically provided by qualified, licensed anesthesia personnel (anesthesiologist, certified nurse anesthetist, or certified anesthesia assistant). The qualified anesthesia provider is trained to monitor and treat the changes in physiologic status associated with sedation, which can bridge into general anesthesia as depth of sedation increases. Anesthesia providers are trained to deal with airway emergencies and have mastery of airway skills. They are also licensed to prescribe and administer vasoactive agents to treat accompanying variances in hemodynamics associated with medication administration at general anesthetic levels of dosing. This factor allows the provider to immediately address complications that arise when infusions and bolus dose medications are administered at anesthetic prescriptive levels.

SUMMARY

Use of pain and sedation scales combined with assessment skills of the RN help guide titration of sedation and pain medications tailored to the patient condition. The RN is crucial to the implementation of targeted light sedation and daily interruption protocols to optimize patient safety and improve patient outcomes. RN-administered sedation is sufficient for much of the patient population; however, there are times when the patient's requirements exceed the amount of sedation medication available to the RN within their scope of practice. During these occasions, when general anesthetic levels of dosing are required, the patient requires an anesthesia provider to facilitate optimal sedation levels.

REFERENCES

1. Barr J, Gilles LF, Puntillo K, et al. Clinical practice guidelines for the management of pain, agitation, and delirium in adult patients in the intensive care unit. Crit Care Med 2013;41(1):263–306.
2. Schelling G, Stoll C, Haller M, et al. Health-related quality of life and posttraumatic stress disorder in survivors of the acute respiratory distress syndrome. Crit Care Med 1998;26:651–9.
3. Granja C, Gomes E, Amaro A, et al, JMIP Study Group. Understanding posttraumatic stress disorder-related symptoms after critical care: the early illness amnesia hypothesis. Crit Care Med 2008;36:2801–9.
4. Stites M. Observational pain scales in critically ill adults. Crit Care Nurse 2013; 33(3):68–78.
5. Puntillo K, Morris A, Thompson C, et al. Pain behaviors observed during six common procedures: results from the Thunder Project II. Crit Care Med 2004;32(2):421–7.
6. Akca O, Melischek M, Scheck T, et al. Postoperative pain and subcutaneous oxygen tension. Lancet 1999;354:41–2.
7. Beilin B, Shavit Y, Hart J, et al. Effects of anesthesia based on large versus small doses of fentanyl on natural killer cell cytotoxicity in the perioperative period. Anesth Analg 1996;82:492–7.
8. Ahlers SJ, van Gulik L, van der Veen AM, et al. Comparison of different pain scoring systems in critically ill patients in a general ICU. Crit Care 2008;12:R15.
9. Fuchs B, Bellamy C. Sedative-analgesic medications in critically ill adults: selection, initiation, maintenance, and withdrawal. In: Parsons PE, Avidan M, Finlay G, editors. UpToDate. Waltham (MA): UpToDate. Accessed July 7, 2014.
10. Riessen R, Pech R, Trankle P, et al. Comparison of the RAMSAY score and the Richmond Agitation Sedation Score: the measurement of sedation depth. Crit Care 2012;16(Suppl 1):P326.

11. Jacobi J, Fraser GL, Coursin DB, et al. Task Force of the American College of Critical Care Medicine (ACCM) of the Society of Critical Care Medicine (SCCM), American Society of Health-System Pharmacists (ASHP), American College of Chest Physicians: clinical practice guidelines for the sustained use of sedatives and analgesics in the critically ill adult. Crit Care Med 2002;30:119–41.
12. Morphine sulfate [package insert]. Eatontown, NJ: Westward Pharmaceuticals; 2011.
13. Hydromorphone hydrochloride [package insert]. Lake Forest, IL: Hospira; 2011.
14. Fentanyl citrate [package insert]. Eatontown, NJ: Westward Pharmaceuticals; 2011.
15. Lexicomp. Fentanyl: drug information. In: UpToDate. Waltham (MA). Accessed July 7, 2014.
16. Midazolam [package insert]. Lake Forest, IL: Hospira; 2012.
17. Bauer TM, Ritz R, Haberthur C, et al. Prolonged sedation due to accumulation of conjugated midazolam. Lancet 1995;346:145–7.
18. Shafer A. Complications of sedation with midazolam in the intensive care unit and a comparison with other sedative regimens. Crit Care Med 1998;26:947–56.
19. Reynolds HN, Teiken P, Regan ME, et al. Hyperlactatemia, increased osmolar gap, and renal dysfunction during continuous lorazepam infusion. Crit Care Med 2000;28:1631–4.
20. Yahwak JA, Riker RR, Fraser GL, et al. Determination of a lorazepam dose threshold for using the osmol gap to monitor for propylene glycol toxicity. Pharmacotherapy 2008;28:984–91.
21. Diprivan (propofol) [package insert]. Schaumburg, IL: APP Pharmaceuticals; 2012.
22. Diedrich DA, Brown DR. Analytic reviews: propofol infusion syndrome in the ICU. J Intensive Care Med 2011;26:59–72.
23. Kam PC, Cardone D. Propofol infusion syndrome. Anaesthesia 2007;62:690–701.
24. Precedex (dexmedetomidine hydrochloride) [package insert]. Lake Forest, IL: Hospira; 2010.
25. Venn RM, Bradshaw CJ, Spencer R, et al. Preliminary UK experience of dexmedetomidine in the surgical patient requiring intensive care. Crit Care 2000;4:302–8.
26. Riker RR, Shehabi Y, Bokesch PM, et al, SEDCOM (Safety and Efficacy of Dexmedetomidine Compared with Midazolam) Study Group. dexmedetomidine vs midazolam for sedation of critically ill patients: a randomized trial. JAMA 2009;301: 489–99.
27. Multz AS. Prolonged dexmedetomidine infusion as an adjunct in treating sedation induced withdrawal. Anesth Analg 2003;96:1054–5.
28. Lexicomp, Inc. Flumazenil: Drug Information. In: UpToDate, Waltham, MA, (Accessed July 7, 2014).
29. Lexicomp. Naloxone: Drug information. In: UpToDate. Waltham (MA). Accessed July 7, 2014.
30. Neumar RW, Otto CW, Link MS, et al. Part 8: adult advanced cardiopulmonary life support: 2010 American Heart Association guidelines for cardiopulmonary resuscitation and emergency cardiovascular care. Circulation 2010;122(18 Suppl 3): 729–67.
31. Gan TJ, Ginsberg B, Glass PS, et al. Opioid-sparing effects of a low-dose infusion of naloxone in patient-administered morphine sulfate. Anesthesiology 1997;87(5): 1075–81.
32. Kress JP, Pohlman AS, O'Connor MF, et al. Daily interruption of sedative infusions in critically ill patients under mechanical ventilation. N Engl J Med 2000;342:1471–7.

33. Girard TD, Kress JP, Fuchs BD, et al. Efficacy and safety of a paired sedation and ventilator weaning protocol for mechanically ventilated patients in intensive care (Awakening and Breathing Controlled Trial): a randomized controlled trial. Lancet 2008;371:126–34.

34. Tanios MA, de Wit M, Epstien SK, et al. Perceived barriers to the use of sedation protocols and daily sedation interruption: a multidisciplinary survey. J Crit Care 2009;24:66–73.

35. Augustes R, Ho KM. Meta-analysis of randomized controlled trials on daily sedation interruption for critically ill adult patients. Anaesth Intensive Care 2011;39(3):401–9.

36. Mehta S, Burry L, Cook D, et al. Daily interruption in mechanically ventilated critically ill patients cared for with a sedation protocol. JAMA 2012;308(19): 1985–92.

37. Hughes CG, Girard TD, Pandharipande PP. Daily sedation interruption versus targeted light sedation strategies in ICU patients. Crit Care Med 2013; 41(Suppl 9):S39–45.

Mechanical Ventilation of the Anesthetized Patient

Nicole K. Damico, CRNA, PhD

KEYWORDS

- Atelectasis • Perioperative • Anesthetized • Continuous mandatory ventilation
- Volume-controlled ventilation • Pressure-controlled ventilation

KEY POINTS

- General anesthesia compromises pulmonary function during the perioperative period.
- A variety of modes and features are now available on the anesthesia ventilator.
- No specific mode or strategy is most effective for all patients and procedures.

INTRODUCTION

Patients who require general anesthesia to undergo a surgical procedure often require mechanical ventilation during the perioperative period. Ventilators incorporated into modern anesthesia machines offer various options for patient management. The unique effects of general anesthesia and surgery on pulmonary physiology must be considered when selecting an individualized plan for mechanical ventilation during the perioperative period. In this article, the pulmonary effects of general anesthesia are reviewed and available options for mechanical ventilation of the anesthetized patient during the perioperative period are presented.

PULMONARY EFFECTS OF GENERAL ANESTHESIA

On assuming care of the patient scheduled for surgery, the anesthesia provider initiates interventions that have unintended negative consequences on pulmonary physiology. Before transferring the patient to the operating room, sedative doses of benzodiazepines in combination with opioids may be given. At low doses, benzodiazepines alone do not cause significant respiratory depression; however, when administered concurrently with opioids, this is more likely.[1] On entering the operating room, the patient is transferred to the operating table in a supine position, with the head of bed flat. The simple act of moving from the upright to a supine position results in a 0.7-L to 0.8-L reduction in functional residual capacity, even in the awake state.[2]

Department of Nurse Anesthesia, School of Allied Health Professions, Virginia Commonwealth University, PO Box 980226, Richmond, VA 23298-0226, USA
E-mail address: damicosn@vcu.edu

Crit Care Nurs Clin N Am 27 (2015) 147–155
http://dx.doi.org/10.1016/j.cnc.2014.10.005
ccnursing.theclinics.com

In anticipation of the period of apnea that often ensues immediately after induction of general anesthesia, it is recommended that patients breathe 100% oxygen by face mask for several minutes or more beforehand. Although preoxygenation extends the period that a patient maintains arterial oxygen saturation in case of prolonged apnea during airway placement,[3] it is also associated with development of absorption atelectasis.[4,5]

The period during which general anesthesia is induced is marked by additional interventions that compromise pulmonary status. Relatively large bolus doses of intravenous sedative/hypnotic agents and narcotics are administered. In combination and at the doses required for this indication, these drugs exert a synergistic effect on pulmonary function, such that induction of general anesthesia frequently results in profound respiratory depression or even periods of apnea.[1] Neuromuscular blockers may also be often given during this period, which induce a state of temporary muscle weakness or complete paralysis. Full support of ventilation is required at the onset of effect of induction drugs. Most often, this support consists of manual positive pressure ventilation by face mask with 100% oxygen via the anesthesia machine breathing circuit and reservoir bag. Assuming the airway is patent, oxygenation and ventilation are effectively supported in the short-term, but can contribute to further development of absorption atelectasis.

Many general anesthetics in the United States are now performed with a laryngeal mask airway (LMA) instead of an endotracheal tube. Muscle relaxation is not required for general anesthetics involving use of an LMA.[6] As a result, increased use of the LMA has resulted in a trend toward allowing patients to breath spontaneously during general anesthesia.[7] Work of breathing during spontaneous ventilation is still significantly increased during spontaneous ventilation through the LMA, albeit less so than during spontaneous ventilation with an endotracheal tube in place.[8]

Whenever muscle relaxant drugs are either not required or their clinical effect has diminished over time, patients breathe spontaneously while under general anesthesia. However, at a level sufficient to permit surgical stimulation, general anesthesia is associated with significant respiratory depression, characterized by irregular respiratory rate and breathing pattern. Pharmacologic agents commonly administered during the maintenance phase of general anesthesia are also associated with a decreased central response to hypercapnia and hypoxia.[4] The effects of anesthetic agents combined with increased work of breathing favor development of atelectasis during extended periods of spontaneous breathing through an artificial airway in the absence of any ventilatory assistance.[7]

PERIOPERATIVE MECHANICAL VENTILATION OPTIONS

The specific modes of mechanical ventilation available on a given anesthesia machine vary by manufacturer, model, and software package installed. In the United States, Dräger (Telford, PA, USA) and GE Healthcare (Wauwatosa, WI) manufacture most anesthesia machines used in clinical practice.[9] It is recommended that anesthesia providers familiarize themselves with the settings and options on the anesthesia machine present at the anesthetizing location before assuming care of the patient. Regardless of manufacturer, anesthesia ventilators are designed and function differently from intensive care unit (ICU) ventilators. These differences are primarily a consequence of the need to contain and properly dispose of respiratory gases, because the anesthesia ventilator serves the dual functions of providing positive pressure support and delivering volatile anesthetic agents. A detailed discussion of anesthesia machine design is beyond the scope of this article. The reader is directed to consult a textbook of anesthesia equipment for additional information.[10] A few of the differences in function between the anesthesia ventilator and the ICU ventilator are discussed.

Continuous Mandatory Ventilation

Continuous mandatory ventilation (CMV) modes are often indicated in the anesthetized patient. General anesthesia at a level sufficient to provide hypnosis, amnesia, analgesia, and areflexia during surgical stimulation is associated with profound respiratory compromise. If an endotracheal tube is inserted, neuromuscular blocking agents are frequently administered to facilitate airway placement under controlled conditions. These agents are intended to create a state of temporary paralysis, such that full ventilator support is needed for the duration of their effect. When the short-acting depolarizing neuromuscular blocker succinylcholine is administered for airway placement, the need for CMV may be only of short duration. Administration of nondepolarizing neuromuscular blockers, either before or after airway placement, necessitates a longer period of full ventilatory support.

In all modes of CMV, the ventilator delivers a breath at set time intervals, irrespective of patient effort. The time interval at which breaths are delivered is determined by setting the respiratory rate. Dividing 1 minute by the respiratory rate, the time allowed for each full ventilator cycle, or 1 cycle of inspiration and exhalation, is determined. The inspiratory/expiratory (I/E) ratio setting dictates the proportion of time during each ventilator cycle allowed for gas delivery and the proportion allowed for passive exhalation. The 2 types of CMV commonly used in the perioperative period are volume-controlled ventilation (VCV) and pressure-controlled ventilation (PCV), which are described here. The range of primary CMV settings available on select anesthesia machines marketed by GE Healthcare and Dräger in the United States is shown in **Table 1**.

Volume-Controlled Ventilation

All modern anesthesia machines can deliver VCV mode. In this form of CMV, the anesthesia provider sets the desired tidal volume. At the preset time, inspiration begins with gas flow from the ventilator rapidly increasing to the rate at which the set tidal volume can be achieved within the inspiratory time allowed. Gas flow then remains at a constant level throughout the inspiratory time. Airway pressure is not controlled during VCV but is instead dependent on airway resistance and pulmonary compliance. As gas flow is initiated at the beginning of the breath, airway pressure increases linearly or exponentially during the inspiratory phase. Pressure-time and flow-time waveforms during VCV are shown in **Fig. 1**. Acute increases in airway resistance or decreases in

Table 1 Anesthesia ventilator settings in VCV and PCV modes				
	Rate (Breaths Per Minute)	I/E Ratio	VCV: Tidal Volume (mL)	PCV: Inspiratory Pressure (cm H_2O)
GE Aespire	4–65	2:1–1:6	45–1500	5–60
GE Aestiva	4–100	2:1–1:8	20–1500	5–50
GE Aisys	4–100	2:1–1:8	20–1500	5–60
GE Avance	4–100	2:1–1:8	20–1500	12–100
Dräger Fabius GS	4–60	4:1–1:4	20–1400	PEEP + 5 ($\leq$70)
Dräger Apollo	3–80	Maximum 5:1	20–1400	PEEP + 5 ($\leq$65)

Abbreviation: PEEP, positive end-expiratory pressure.

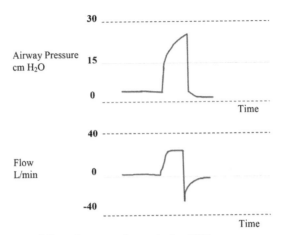

Fig. 1. Pressure-time and flow-time waveforms during VCV.

airway compliance can result in excessive airway pressures during VCV. As a safety mechanism, the anesthesia machine is equipped with a pressure limit (P_{lim} or P_{max}) setting, which allows the provider to set the maximum pressure delivered to the patient.

VCV is suitable for patients of all ages and acuity levels. Once a concern when providing anesthesia to neonates and infants, recent advances in anesthesia ventilator design now enable accurate delivery of low tidal volumes in VCV mode across a wide range of lung compliances.[11] The major advantage of VCV is that minute ventilation is guaranteed. Another advantage is the ability to ensure that excessive tidal volume is not delivered to the patient inadvertently, thereby reducing the risk of ventilator-induced lung injury.[12]

Pressure-Controlled Ventilation

Many anesthesia ventilators now offer PCV (**Fig. 2**). This mode requires the anesthesia provider to set the desired inspiratory pressure level ($P_{INSPIRED}$ or P_{INSP}). As a form of CMV, machine breaths in PCV are initiated and ended at the preset time interval,

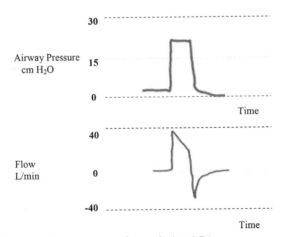

Fig. 2. Pressure-time and flow-time waveforms during PCV.

without regard to patient effort. At the onset of inspiration, gas flows into the breathing circuit, until the inspiratory pressure target is achieved. Anesthesia ventilators permit manual adjustment of the rate of pressure increase during PCV. Once the target pressure is reached, pressure in the circuit and the pressure in the alveoli begin to equilibrate, such that the rate of gas flow needed to maintain the set pressure level decreases throughout inspiration. This pattern of gas flow generates a characteristic decelerating pattern on the flow-time waveform and a square curve on the pressure-time waveform, as shown in **Fig. 2**. Delivered tidal volume is not controlled in PCV but is instead dependent on airway resistance and compliance.

PCV can be safely applied in patients of all ages and acuity levels. The most significant disadvantage in the perioperative period is that contextual factors can cause abrupt changes in respiratory impedance. With acute increases in airway resistance or decreases in compliance, the delivered tidal volume may not be sufficient to provide adequate minute ventilation. Conversely, with acute decreases in compliance, such as on release of gas pneumoperitoneum at the end of a laparoscopic procedure, excessive tidal volume can be inadvertently delivered to the patient.

Dual-Controlled Modes: The Best of Both Worlds?

Some anesthesia ventilators offer the ability to deliver gas flow in a decelerating pattern as in PCV while also guaranteeing tidal volume delivery as in VCV. On ventilators manufactured by GE Healthcare, this quality is called "pressure-controlled ventilation with volume guaranteed (PCV-VG)." Dräger refers to this mode as "volume mode autoflow (volume AF)." In either case, the anesthesia provider sets the desired tidal volume, respiratory rate, I/E ratio, and P_{max}. The ventilator delivers an initial volume-controlled breath at a constant flow rate, enabling determination of the patient's compliance. All subsequent machine breaths are delivered with a decelerating flow pattern at the inspiratory pressure level required to deliver the set tidal volume, given the patient's calculated compliance. With each subsequent breath, compliance is recalculated, and the inspiratory pressure level is automatically adjusted for by as much as ± 3 cm H_2O to maintain consistent tidal volume delivery. **Fig. 3** shows pressure-time and flow-time waveforms during this mode. Note the initial VCV breath and obvious change to PCV for the second breath.

Synchronized Intermittent Mandatory Ventilation

Synchronized intermittent mandatory ventilation (SIMV) is hybrid mode of mechanical ventilation available only on select anesthesia ventilators. This mode provides

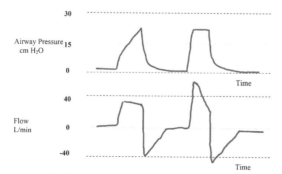

Fig. 3. Pressure-time and flow-time waveforms during initiation of dual-triggered controlled mechanical ventilation.

guaranteed minimum volume delivery and allows the patient to determine when breaths are delivered. Unlike in the ICU, SIMV is often used as a safety net rather than a weaning strategy during the perioperative period. In case of unanticipated abrupt changes in the patient's respiratory pattern, such as in response to a bolus dose of an opioid or a change in the inhaled anesthetic agent concentration, SIMV provides a minimum number of mandatory breaths. The ventilator attempts to synchronize these breaths with spontaneous effort by the patient, if present. When the patient is apneic, the ventilator delivers the minimum number of machine breaths only. Spontaneous respiratory effort between machine breaths generates gas flow to the patient, unlike in CMV modes. Another notable difference between SIMV and CMV modes is that the duration of the inspiratory time during machine breaths is determined by directly setting the inspiratory time in seconds rather than the I/E ratio.

Other key parameters should be set on the anesthesia ventilator in SIMV mode. The first is the trigger level. Most anesthesia ventilators are flow triggered, with the trigger level therefore selected as a value in liters per minute. The trigger window setting refers to the time during which the ventilator monitors for spontaneous respiratory attempts to synchronize the next machine breath. Trigger window is selected as a percentage of the expiratory time measured backwards from the next mandatory breath, with possible values in the range 0% to 80%. When the patient's spontaneous effort generates inspiratory flow that is (1) at a rate that exceeds the trigger level and (2) timed within the trigger window; a synchronized machine breath is initiated. Adjustments in the trigger level and trigger window settings can achieve optimal patient-ventilator synchrony.

Mandatory breaths in SIMV mode on the anesthesia ventilator may be volume controlled or pressure controlled, dependent on the manufacturer, model, and software package installed. The parameter to be controlled must be set as appropriate for the mode. That is, if the mode is volume controlled, tidal volume must be selected, and if the mode is pressure controlled, the inspiratory pressure level must be set. Anesthesia ventilators also offer the option to provide pressure support during spontaneous breaths in combination with SIMV.

Pressure Support Ventilation

Newer anesthesia ventilators offer pressure support ventilation (PSV) as a stand-alone mode or as an optional setting during use of SIMV. PSV during the perioperative period may be used for weaning indications or to offset the pulmonary effects of general anesthesia during extended periods of spontaneous breathing with an artificial airway in place.[7] PSV may also be used alone or in combination with expiratory support in the form of positive end-expiratory pressure (PEEP) via face mask during the perioperative period. Application of this strategy improves the effectiveness of preoxygenation in patients who are at high risk of postinduction desaturation, such as the morbidly obese,[13] thereby creating a larger margin of safety during airway management.

PSV provides inspiratory augmentation during spontaneous respiratory efforts. Machine assistance is flow triggered on most anesthesia ventilators, meaning that gas flow is initiated when the patient generates inspiratory flow exceeding the set trigger level in liters per minute. The rate of gas flow increases until the set inspiratory pressure level is reached. Some anesthesia ventilators permit the user to manually adjust the rate of gas flow, or the rate of increase, in PSV. As in other pressure-targeted modes of mechanical ventilation, gas flow rate then automatically decreases throughout inspiration, as is possible while maintaining the set inspiratory pressure level.

A reasonable initial setting for the inspiratory pressure level in PSV mode is in the range of 5 to 10 cm H_2O. The ideal inspiratory pressure level is the minimum necessary to achieve an appropriate tidal volume during pressure-supported breaths. The frequent need for adjustments in the anesthetic level during an operative procedure often causes wide variations in the respiratory pattern and the potential for periods of apnea. Accordingly, anesthesia ventilators are equipped with a unique setting that ensures a minimum respiratory rate during use of PSV. GE Healthcare trademarked the name PSVPro to refer to pressure support with apnea backup. GE ventilators equipped with PSVPro require the anesthesia provider to set a backup respiratory rate of at least 2 breaths per minute (bpm). Dräger refers to the backup rate setting as the minimum frequency in PSV mode, which can be turned off or set at a minimum of 3 bpm. Whenever the backup rate is needed, regardless of manufacturer, machine breaths are delivered as in SIMV mode.

Pressure-supported breaths on the anesthesia ventilator may be flow cycled or time cycled, which refers to the parameter that determines when machine support is terminated during augmented breaths. If flow cycled, gas flow is discontinued when the inspiratory flow rate declines lower than the level set by the anesthesia provider. This level may be expressed as a percentage of the maximum inspiratory flow achieved during the breath (range 5%–50%) or as a discrete flow rate in liters per minute. Time-cycled anesthesia ventilators terminate gas flow after the set inspiratory time, in seconds, is achieved.

Continuous Positive Airway Pressure

Few anesthesia machines offer continuous positive airway pressure as a ventilator mode. This form of support is available on any anesthesia machine if the patient is connected to the anesthesia machine breathing circuit using a face mask or artificial airway to create a closed system and the selector switch on the machine is turned to the manual ventilation position. Manual adjustment of the adjustable pressure limit valve allows positive pressure to generate in the breathing system at the pressure level the anesthesia provider deems appropriate for the patient and situation.

Positive End-Expiratory Pressure

PEEP is typically available on the anesthesia ventilator. Newer anesthesia machines have an integrated electronically controlled PEEP valve.[10] Dräger anesthesia machines can be set to deliver PEEP 0 to 20 cm H_2O in 1 cm H_2O increments. On GE Healthcare anesthesia machines, the provider can opt to turn PEEP off or select a value in the range of 4 to 30 cm H_2O, in 1 cm H_2O increments.

Selection of Strategies for Perioperative Mechanical Ventilation

The plan for mechanical ventilation during the perioperative period must be individualized. Factors in determining the most appropriate strategy include the patient's medical history, planned method of airway management, anesthetic technique, planned procedure, positioning requirements, and the features available on the anesthesia ventilator at hand. Situations in which mechanical ventilation can be completely avoided during general anesthesia are rare, such as a short procedure for which muscle relaxation is not required, and a lighter level of general anesthesia is sufficient to prevent reaction to the surgical stimulus. The composite effect of anesthetic agents, adjunct medications, surgical stress, positioning, and environmental factors has such a significant impact on pulmonary physiology that mechanical ventilation of some variation is often advisable.[7] When CMV modes are indicated during the perioperative period, no particular mode of ventilation has been consistently shown to be clinically superior for certain procedures or patient populations.[14] It is more important to properly select and customize parameters within whatever mode is utilized. The intraoperative period is unique, in that it is often marked by acute changes in the patient's status secondary to factors such as varying levels of surgical stimulation, administration of bolus doses of anesthetic medications, acute blood loss, or dramatic changes in patient position (or the operating table position). Incremental changes in mechanical ventilation settings are therefore required at more frequent intervals than in other patient care areas.

Goals for oxygenation and ventilation of the anesthetized patient are no different than for the mechanically ventilated patient in other patient care areas. It is standard of care to continuously monitor pulse oximetry during any anesthetic. In general, maintaining an arterial oxygen saturation at 90% or greater is sufficient to meet oxygen demand during the perioperative period.[15] Exhaled carbon dioxide is also monitored continuously whenever artificial airway support is provided.[16,17] End-tidal carbon dioxide (ET_{CO_2}) levels are generally 2 to 5 mm Hg lower than the partial pressure of carbon dioxide in arterial blood (Pa_{CO_2}).[10] To maintain a normal Pa_{CO_2} of 35 to 45 mm Hg, adjustments in mechanical ventilation settings are therefore often targeted to maintain ET_{CO_2} between 30 and 40 mm Hg.

The anesthesia ventilator is equipped with monitors of airway pressure, volume, and flow. As in the ICU, these parameters are valuable for determining appropriate adjustments in ventilator settings during the perioperative period. Airway pressure parameters, which may include PEEP, mean airway pressure, peak airway pressure, or plateau pressure, are shown on a small screen on the anesthesia ventilator display panel as a numeric value in cm/H_2O. Most anesthesia ventilators also show airway pressure graphically as a pressure-time waveform by default. Software graphic packages that show respiratory spirometry loops are available on some newer anesthesia machines.[10] Arterial blood gas analysis is performed on an as needed basis to guide patient management in complex situations.

SUMMARY/DISCUSSION

Anesthetized patients are at risk of pulmonary compromise during the perioperative period. The effects of general anesthesia and a myriad of other context-specific factors represent a unique indication for mechanical ventilation support. Selection of an appropriate strategy for mechanical ventilation of the anesthetized patient must account for all of the relevant patient and contextual factors. Modern anesthesia ventilators have a variety of modes and options that can be used to provide safe and effective ventilatory support to the anesthetized patient during the perioperative period.

REFERENCES

1. Stoelting RK, Hillier SC. Pharmacology & physiology in anesthetic practice. 4th edition. Philadelphia: Lippincott Williams & Wilkins; 2006.
2. Wahba RW. Perioperative functional residual capacity. Can J Anaesth 1991;38: 384–400.
3. Weingart SD, Levitan RM. Preoxygenation and prevention of desaturation during emergency airway management. Ann Emerg Med 2012;59(3):165–75.
4. Hedenstierna G. Respiratory physiology. In: Miller RD, Eriksson LI, editors. Miller's anesthesia. 7th edition. Philadelphia: Churchill Livingstone/Elsevier; 2010. p. 381.
5. Duggan M, Kavanaugh BP. Pulmonary atelectasis: a pathogenic perioperative entity. Anesthesiology 2005;102:838–54.

6. Verghese C, Mena G, Ferson DZ, et al. Laryngeal mask airway. In: Hagberg CA, editor. Benumof and Hagberg's airway management. 3rd edition. Philadelphia: Churchill Livingstone/Elsevier; 2013. p. 468.

7. Magnusson L, Docent P. Role of spontaneous and assisted ventilation during general anesthesia. Best Pract Res Clin Anaesthesiol 2010;24:243–52.

8. Joshi GP, Morrison SG, White PF, et al. Work of breathing in anesthetized patients: laryngeal mask airway versus tracheal tube. J Clin Anesth 1998;10:268–71.

9. Dosch M. The anesthesia gas machine 2012. Available at: http://www.udmercy. edu/crna/agm/. Accessed August 18, 2014.

10. Dorsch JA, Dorsch SE, editors. Understanding anesthesia equipment. 5th edition. Philadelphia: Lippincott Williams & Wilkins; 2008.

11. Bachiller PR, McDonough JM, Feldman JM. Do new anesthesia ventilators deliver small tidal volumes accurately during volume-controlled ventilation? Anesth Analg 2008;106(5):1392–400.

12. Slutsky AS, Ranieri VM. Ventilator-induced lung injury. N Engl J Med 2013; 369(22):2126–36.

13. Delay J, Sebbane M, Jung B, et al. The effectiveness of noninvasive positive pressure ventilation to enhance preoxygenation in morbidly obese patients: a randomized controlled study. Anesth Analg 2008;107(5):1707–13.

14. Aguilar G, Belda FJ, Badenes R, et al. Ventilatory pressure modes in anesthesia. Curr Anaesth Crit Care 2010;21:255–61.

15. Warner MA, Patel B. Mechanical ventilation. In: Hagberg CA, editor. Benumof and Hagberg's airway management. 3rd edition. Philadelphia: Churchill Livingstone/ Elsevier; 2013. p. 984.

16. American Association of Nurse Anesthetists. Standards for nurse anesthesia practice. 2013. Available at: http://www.aana.com/resources2/professionalpractice/ Pages/Standards-for-Nurse-Anesthesia-Practice.aspx. Accessed August 30, 2014.

17. American Society of Anesthesiologists, Standards and Practice Parameters Committee. Standards for basic anesthetic monitoring. 2011. Available at: https://www.asahq.org/For-Members/Standards-Guidelines-and-Statements.aspx. Accessed August 28, 2014.

Printed and bound by CPI Group (UK) Ltd, Croydon, CR0 4YY

07/10/2024

01040499-0017